"Life, like art, is not a thing but rather offers ways of seeing and savoring. In *Pies to Die For*, you'll be challenged to grapple with your mortality and fragility. You'll be invited to feel more deeply, to think more expansively, and to value the willingness to wonder in new ways.

Whether or not you're a cancer survivor or cancer patient, you'll be richer and wiser for having experienced the stories and experiences this book offers."

—Sheila Pearl, MSW, CLC
Relationship & Recalibration Life Coach
Author of Amazon Bestselling *Ageless & Sexy* book series

"Cancer is an overwhelming and unwelcome interloper. In light of its seemingly insurmountable power, those who are condemned to its diagnosis so often—if not universally—feel helpless and powerless. Thankfully Carole Weaver's *Pies to Die For* is a source of hope in what would otherwise be a dark existence.

Dr. Weaver doesn't downplay or avoid the Herculean challenges that a cancer diagnosis entails. Rather, she shines much-needed light on a road that takes you away from the endless spiral of depression and death to a place of hope and positivity. A place of life.

Anyone suffering with cancer or a similar diagnosis must read this book for their own well-being and, most fundamentally, for their happiness."

— Jeff Neurman
blood

D1490536

"To read Carole Weaver is to love her. This follow-up to her luminous *Side Effects* is another delightful perspective shifter. Refusing to submit to the maudlin and morose, Carole introduces us to an enchanting array of people and scenarios she and her husband, Ken (an antiques and art appraiser), have encountered.

In an era where confusion and tumult reign, Carole exposes the light, the beauty, and the sheer joy of living, encouraging gratitude and optimism in her readers."

—**Tracey S. Lawrence**
Author, *Dementia Sucks: A Caregiver's Journey –
With Lessons Learned*

"Carole Weaver shares a profound journey in *Pies to Die For*, an exploration of how experiencing the aesthetic can lead to deep human emotional healing. Here lies the resources that are a gift for anyone dealing with a severe diagnosis. We are not alone in our grief when we see how its' simultaneity can be a means to befriend it, opening the energy of compassion and humor to deal with it."

—**Dr. Kenneth Silvestri**
Author, *A Wider Lens: How to See Your Life Differently*

"This book is not only a primer for those with THE DIAGNOSIS, it's a primer for living a full life. More than that, this book is a testament to the author's love of life."

—**Lynn J. Maier**, Esquire

"How lucky we are to have this brilliant author share her stories with us! Through stage four metastatic cancer, Dr. Weaver delivers five-star inspiration.

—Dr. Jandie Schwartz
University of Pittsburgh Medical Center,
Co-leader of the Breast Cancer Book Club

"*In Pies to Die For,* Carole Weaver brilliantly injects a rare positivity and patina into the fabric of Metastatic Breast Cancer (MBC). She weaves her magic throughout this mesmerizing narrative, using quaint, anecdotal sequences that seamlessly delineate the grief of an MBC diagnosis as 'water falling into a cistern with no light.'"

—Laura Carfang, EdD
Executive Director & Founder, Survivingbreastcancer.
Org

In my years of dealing with serious illness—as a patient, a writer, and as a medical musician—I've never met anyone who knows how to deal with it in a better way than Carole Weaver. She's a marvel and an inspiration. This book, beautifully written, is a must-read for anyone and everyone who is touched by life-threatening illness.

—Andrew Schulman
Author, *Waking the Spirit: A Musician's Journey Healing Body, Mind, and Soul*

PIES TO
DIE FOR

PIES TO DIE FOR

HOW TO LIVE A VIBRANT LIFE DESPITE A FATAL DIAGNOSIS

CAROLE WEAVER, PhD

Stonebrook Publishing
Saint Louis, Missouri

A STONEBROOK PUBLISHING BOOK
Copyright ©2021 Carole Weaver-Linsner

This book was guided in development and
edited by Nancy L. Erickson, The Book Professor®
TheBookProfessor.com

Library of Congress Control Number: 2021902355

ISBN: 978-1-7358021-7-6

www.stonebrookpublishing.net

DEDICATION

For Ken—
and for all those coping with a serious illness, especially
Teryn McKewin, beloved sister-in-law and friend.

CONTENTS

PREFACE

It is the water of the Caribbean that I love most of all—tepid or flesh warm, the color is divine. I always wanted a turquoise convertible, probably because it would be so lovely to drive around and pretend I was in the sea I craved.

My favorite beach on Saint Martin is the so-called nude beach on the French side. Orient Beach, the place where you could be sure to see the naked ladies sunning themselves. My husband, Ken, sometimes took surreptitious photos of the topless tanned ladies. The Titty Project. Even after I lost a breast to cancer in 2007, I didn't mind the voyeurism. I was healthy and life was good.

At Orient Beach, the sea stretches out before you in all its turquoise glory. This is actually the Atlantic, although it is fed by the Caribbean. There you will find, only occasionally, some wave action reminiscent of my childhood in Ocean City, Maryland, where, if you were not careful, you could be knocked down by the strength of the Atlantic curl, or even dragged out to sea by the undertow. But the Caribbean islands are not known for these surfer waves. I was used to the placidity of the gorgeous color, the clarity of the water.

That day, it surprised me, the waves at Orient. They were almost muscular, and I felt the water hurl my body, and then one slammed me down to the sand.

This was the beginning of the pain in my back.

It was also the time of my first grandchild's birth. While I was on vacation in the Caribbean the first week of February, he was born on February 6, 2016, in Los Angeles, California. The phone call to the resort a few miles from Orient Beach came in the middle of the night. Sleepless that night while I listened to the sea outside, I was waiting for it.

"You have a grandson, Mom," my younger son, David, said.

"Oh my God, how wonderful. Everybody well?" I asked.

"Yes! And his name is McKewin Weaver, named after granddad."

A thrilling surprise that brought so much joy! McKewin was my maiden name. My father's nickname was "Mac." He had died forty-two years before. Mac never saw either of his grandsons, James and David. How moved I was: my oldest son and his wife named their firstborn after him. Mac Weaver had come into the world with a salute to his great-grandfather.

When I got home to New York a week later, the pain in my back had become excruciating. At the airport in Saint Martin while we waited for the airplane, I was in such distress that another traveler, who looked like she knew about mind-altering drugs, offered me a pill from her extensive portable pharmacopeia:

"Here, honey. It looks like you're in a bad way."

"Oh, no, I couldn't. I take blood pressure pills," I objected.

"That don't make no difference." She shook her platinum hair and pressed the little plastic box toward me.

"That plane is late and it's gonna be a while . . ." she continued. "This is Darvocet. Harmless. I had a bad back for years. With this stuff, now I can stand it."

I stared at the white round button, not jagged at all. Not the way I felt, the pain cutting my lower back like a rusty saber in the hands of a madman.

"Well, do you think it will be OK?" My hands were shaking around the water bottle while I gulped down the offering. Gratefully.

Here was a real character: clearly high—and wealthy. Most of her utterances didn't make sense, but she knew what agony looked like. I took down her contact information and despite my e-mailed thank you, I never heard from her again.

At home in New York, when I went to the local health clinic, I was glad to see the nice nurse practitioner, Ashley, who had earlier given me my flu shot. She examined me and, with her eyes averting mine, called my cardiologist who ordered a CAT scan.

When Ashley called with the news, it was two days before I was to leave for my important trip to Los Angeles to meet my new grandson.

"You have cancer cells in your lung and lower back," blurted the voice on the other end of the phone.

The room went cold and disbelief shot through me like an injection of ice. *Must be the wrong person attached to the wrong test*, I thought. But it WAS Ashley's voice. She said my name with a little tremor.

"But I have a grandson I must see in California. My first grandson."

She ignored the non-sequitur, pausing for a moment. Then she urged me to give her the name of my former oncologist, Dr. T, whom I hadn't seen in years. He would be sent the results and then I would know more.

The shock bent my head over the phone. I'd had breast cancer nine years before, an ordeal I preferred to forget: the infections, the chemo, the surgeries. But I took Arimedex to control the estrogen, the trigger for my type of cancer, and for five years after the last visit to Dr. T, I'd enjoyed one of the happiest chapters of my life. Here it was, years after I saw him for the last time. While I enjoyed my life and looked away, could it be? The horrible pain in my back was a herald. The Monster was back. With a vengeance.

I was still determined to get on the plane, and when I got to LA, confirm the diagnosis.

LOS ANGELES, MARCH 2016, THE MRI

Boom boomboomboomboom eeeee ahahahaH BOOM uhuhuh boomboomboom bangbangbangBANG

The cylinders turned with horror. The doctors confirmed the findings of the scan taken a month earlier in New York. I had tumors in my spine and lungs, probably from the breast cancer I survived nine years before. Metastatic. The syllables of the word conjured Halloween, and they screamed that the life I knew was over.

The drumming went on incessantly for thirty minutes, the sound surely of hell's greeting; an incantation meant for the mad; or the perfect instrument to drive you there.

"Don't move," said the attendant. "Now, breathe, breathe. DON'T BREATHE!"

Outside the Imaging Center was the City of Dreams, the edges of Hollywood where my sons were successful in the movie industry. I was 3,000 miles from my home in a wild contradiction: the first sight of my first grandchild and the start of my treatment for stage four cancer, both at the same time. New life in the midst of death foretold.

—◦◦◦—

Ken and I had only been married eight years on that MRI morning in 2016. Ours was a surprising ignition of a love affair that marked the end of my twenty-plus years of single parenting.

In 2005, I worked in a New York suburb; my sons were out of college and living in California. And I was ready for Broadway. At sixty-two, I was encouraged by my directors in amateur musical theatre to try out for those bit parts for older women who wear gaudy costumes and stay upstage in plays like *Sweeny Todd*; or, even sometimes, downstage, in a starring role, like the Elaine Stritch part in *Company*, singing:

"Here's to the ladies who lunch, everybody laugh. Lounging in their kaftans and planning a lunch on their own behalf . . . I'll drink to that!"

Since college forty years earlier, and for the last few years, I had smelled enough greasepaint to yearn for the boards of the theatres on the Great White Way under my feet. I wanted to wail with a smokey voice the tunes of Sondheim, or even listen as an extra.

But it was either a miracle or the operations of a loving ghost who interrupted my Broadway melody and made my meeting with Ken possible.

Several years before, in 2002, I was listening to the end of a psychic's reading in Nyack, New York. Her insights that my employer's board of directors was a confused bunch certainly turned out to be true; that my sons were good-hearted, but not always forthright; and that when I was too compassionate about the suffering of others, I should hold my head on the right side to recover—these all struck valid and helpful chords. I felt content with the world of prophecy and psychic vision and got ready to leave.

I paid Litany her fee and turned toward the door when she stopped me.

"Someone named Mac is here," she said. My hand froze on the doorknob.

"Mac?" Litany frowned, trying to understand something. "He is saying something . . . can't quite get it."

"That's my father's name, Mac McKewin. He'd died in 1974—and suddenly—of a heart attack to my ravaging grief and loss."

Litany listened to something hard to hear.

After a long pause, she said, "Here is what he is saying: 'He's coming . . . don't worry . . . he's coming.'"

"Who's coming?" I asked. "Daddy?"

Litany said, "I don't think he means himself."

Still confused, I left her office.

Three years passed and no visitation from Daddy, so I forgot about it.

I was a full-time fund raiser at a women's college. I fit in my musical comedy hobby in the evenings and weekends.

One day in the office the phone rang, a call from Contessa Blavia Lotti Wondola, my biggest donor at the time. She had just given the college a promise of $100,000 in her will—a generous legacy. Still, the most revocable of gifts need care and feeding of the donor lest they change their mind.

"Dr. Weaver, you must help me. I purchased a $20,000 table at a fund-raiser tomorrow night and one of my guests took ill. Won't you go to fill in the table?"

"Tomorrow night?" I squeaked. She knew the production was dark that evening. I had conflicting visions of a night of much-needed rest from the role of Fraulein Schneider in *Cabaret* with my feet up to watch *Jeopardy* versus the $100,000 legacy floating away with the Contessa's disappointed face.

The following night, I barely made the seven o'clock train bound for Grand Central and the famous Sky Club on the 56th floor. In those days, The Sky Club was up the escalator in the great hall and up again to the top floor of the then-Pan Am Building. Windows surrounded the dining room and they looked out on the greatest city in the world; but that view was rivalled by a stunning collection of paintings and a spectacular mural of ports of the world on all the walls.

Tall, silver-haired Irish Catholic males in tuxedos, most of them more rich than religious, made my fund-raiser's heart sing. But I knew I had to find the Contessa, meet my table companions, charm the company, and leave as soon as grace allowed.

No Contessa. She was late, and I was becoming a little bored with strangers saying with conceit, "I work for the Holy See—that is, the Vatican." I chatted with a judge, and then turned to face a hallway with a red carpet.

At the end of it was a man who seemed as if he had just caught sight of me and was about to speak. Here was another silver-haired gentleman in a tuxedo, but with a long, red silk scarf around the collar—a beautiful, original touch. The scarf and the rug and his smile pulled me, so I walked the twelve feet to his side and said,

"I'm Dr. Weaver from the College, and who are you?"

"I'm Ken Linsner, and I'm the curator for all this art. The Sky Club will close in a few weeks, and the collection must go to auction."

"Well," I said, "How intriguing . . . Tell me about this portrait."

"This is a famous eighteenth-century artist . . ." he began.

He was brilliant, fascinating, and later that night, he asked if I would like to go to a Russian photography exhibit the following Tuesday. I said yes that I spoke a little Russian, and we exchanged cards just before his escort arrived to stare daggers at me.

He never called, so by Friday, I felt obsessed, and did what I never do: I called *him*. I sensed that this man would change my life, and, although the courtship that followed was certainly bumpy—I listened to my heart, not my head.

It was days, maybe weeks after the Sky Club meeting that I realized that the night I met Ken was November 9, the anniversary of my father's death. "He's coming," Mac had said years earlier at the psychic.

"He's coming"—Ken, the love of my life and the blessing that was better than Broadway.

—◦◦◦—

Ashley's phone call destroyed the near decade of renewal, adventure, ripening mature love, and apparent health and energy.

The Phone Call: overwhelming. Colossal sense of loss, of peace of mind, of trust in the future, of plans. All vanished. *Before* and *after* The Call. My life cut in half. Grief, unbearable grief. The knife ready to strike, thrusting in the air above my head.

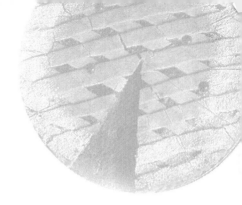

1

GRIEF

*And when [grief] comes, it's a bow-down . . . And it comes when
it wants to, and it carves you out—it comes in the middle of the
night, comes in the middle of the day, comes in the middle of a
meeting, comes in the middle of a meal. It arrives.*

—Elizabeth Gilbert

GRIEF PART ONE

The emotion of grief has always conjured images of
magnificent art forms for me. Michelangelo's *Pietà*
with the Mother holding her dead thirty-three-
year-old son, her head bowed over his body recalling other
Madonnas, especially maternal arms around the baby Jesus.
Now a tragic reprise: her collapsed posture and her barely

visible face under her hood as she gazes at the grown man across her lap—and holds us in ineffable sadness.

Grief is also brilliantly explored and rendered by the New York Memorial for 9/11. The huge square fountain is comprised of walls of water running down each of the four sides to a central shallow lake and then to a deeper smaller cistern, black and foreboding. The light never shines in this square hole. The sound of water silences even the most cheerful tourists who walk up to the memorial's outer square border. The sight moves me for its magnificent metaphor of tears, the depth of loss, the ongoing energy of keening, of remembering what is gone. And when you stop to look, your hands lean on the names carved into the slanted border. It is shiny copper, and your palms have the vague sense of being cut. The letters of the names shout with irresistible definition, the loudest noise on the scene, floating above the sound of running water.

The grief of the discovery that you might die sooner than you hoped, expected; that your length of life is surely endangered by stage four cancer—this is a paralyzing thought that never quite leaves you. It only can be pushed away, sometimes shoved back by a better PET scan or blood test, or your doctor's reminder that the cancer is stable, or a story of one who lived ten years after the diagnosis.

But it never leaves—it is the sound of water falling into a cistern with no light.

At first, I wept a lot in various churches and on my pillow when I was visiting family in Los Angeles without Ken. When you cry that hard, it is a terrible ache, but it purges and purifies. The sound of that cry is, like Mark Nepo says, a kind of song. A terrible song, but a song, nonetheless.

When I was finished crying, I looked around.
Then I wanted to know how other people grieved.

The grief of the discovery that you might die sooner than you hoped, expected; that your length of life is surely endangered by stage four cancer—this is a paralyzing thought that never quite leaves you.

So, the way people handle sorrow this deep was what I thought about when Ken told me the story of the $15,000 bed in a double-wide trailer.

He was called on to appraise the damages of the insured furniture for the client. *A $15,000 bed in a double wide?* he thought. In a walker, the woman greeted him at the door and brought him to a large bed shoved into a smallish room. A gunshot smashed the headboard and damaged the bed's marble side tables.

"Yeah, it sure is a mess, right? That's what a 38-caliber revolver will do to fine wood," she said. "Uh course, the worse of it is that gun killed Jake, my son. He had been downhearted for weeks. Didn't even get out of bed most days."

Ken stopped measuring the hole in the headboard and turned to her. "Your son shot himself here?"

Woman said, "Right. Shot himself in the head, my only boy."

She did not weep. Ken only remembered her twisted face, insistent presence, and non-stop chatter, while he took pictures to determine the price of the repair of the bed or the amount State Farm would give the woman for a settlement.

Despite her loss and the remembrance, it seemed that she wanted the bed fixed.

After his work, Ken felt a bit shaken by the experience and decided to go into the small town for some refreshment. It was a strange, unpeopled village. The hotel looked like something from the old TV show *Gunsmoke*, and the library was about as big as a latrine. Only one store looked lively. He walked in and met the owner who was so glad to see Ken that he engaged him in excited conversation. Ken asked him about the suicide and the baker said that the son, in his twenties, had become depressed because he could not get work. He stole the suicide gun from his mother's boyfriend who was there frequently.

But the baker really wanted to talk about his pastry genius and the "made-from-scratch" deliciousness of his products. Ken bought a strawberry rhubarb pie to bring home to me.

When he left the shop, he turned to see the name of the store: **PIES TO DIE FOR.**

Here was a concept to live by if you are confronting a terminal illness: a fascinating and somehow comforting philosophy that combines something luscious with death itself. Leslie Jamieson comes close to it in an interview when she describes her favorite thing to read. It is about "acute simultaneity"—how life can give us—and at the same time—wonder and weirdness; beauty and danger; vitality and mortality.

Accepting this mixed bag is important for people who are determined to live with vigor and joy along with the knowledge that we may not have much time left to do just that.

It is no easy trick to handle the diagnosis—to be alive and yet know there is no cure. To be in love with life, with our darlings, and recognize an ending could be near. Acute simultaneity—how do we accept this awful paradox and savor magic and magnificence while we can? How do we practice what H. L. Mencken suggested: "We cannot make our life longer. But we can make it wider."

A wider life, I surmise, looks for wisdom in the way others face loss. I have embraced that search in my husband's clients.

Ken creates appraisals for those who have lost art through death, debt, divorce, or disaster. Let's look at each situation. Clients will ask to formally evaluate their art for their estate, so that the IRS will know, for tax purposes, what has been transferred to family or charitable institutions or friends when they pass on. Appraisals are also needed for insurance companies. Insurance will "cover," for example, art that has been damaged or destroyed when an official appraisal is submitted. Flooding and fire, building collapse, and other forces of destruction result in either repair or remuneration to the owner.

Also, in order to save their financial predicament, clients will ask Ken to estimate value so the art can be sold. Divorce often requires that the art, like all possessions, is somehow divided between spouses. The law requires an official appraisal for the division.

Sometimes the situation of lost or damaged art teaches us a lesson about the kind of loss we are facing—our health, our peace of mind, our plans for the future, our joy, even our identity—the art form of our lives. Sometimes, it teaches us how NOT to deal with loss.

—✦—

We will never know how the woman with the dead son handled the closure of her grief. Incessant talk was her version of "sharing her pain" with friends or counselors—even to Ken, the stranger who came from the insurance company. Expressing the hurt is one of the easements of grief. Accepting the reality of loss, according to J.W. Worden, working through the pain, and adjusting to life, and then moving on. Or, as many prefer, Kubler-Ross's Five stages of grief: denial, anger, bargaining, depression, and acceptance. You will find some of these stages addressed in this book.

However, facing a death of a loved one is different from receiving a diagnosis that signals death for yourself. For me, the numbness that accompanied my first weeks in grief was probably a good thing. As Elizabeth Gilbert tells us, we have no power over grief. It takes over physically, and we must humbly let it bow us down. Yet, the early stage of grief gave me time to get a clearer sense of what my options were, which doctors to engage, where to be treated, and what kind of medication I should take.

For me, the single most important power punch to get the heavy load of grief off my chest was holding my first grandson in my arms, only a few weeks after the gate-to-hell phone call.

I have a picture of myself in a chair with Mac Weaver bundled in my arms. I can barely look at my face because it is so contorted in crying, in coping with one of the first moments of acute simultaneity. The miracle of that little creature, who stared up at me and smelled like vanilla and just-cut grass, lifted the sorrow and made me angry at the same time. The moment told me that I *must* live to see him grow—even if it meant only to be there a little longer—so he might know me. I must find a way to bolster my life force, fight the pain in my back, the growing cancer, and get the time to let him understand that I love him so.

For me, the single most important power punch to get the heavy load of grief off my chest was holding my first grandson in my arms, only a few weeks after the gate-to-hell phone call.

Today, four years later, he is still 3,000 miles away, but there have been delicious visits when I could tell him about Hercules and then watch the Disney movie together, cuddled on the couch under an afghan. And then there is FaceTime and texts and phones and airplanes and packages for me to send to him with toys and books and costumes of superheroes he can wear (for he has his grandmother's theatrical sense.) But there are, most of all, airplanes. I love airplanes I can get on.

So, the first antidote to my grief was my becoming a grandmother and holding that child. The second came from the head oncologist at Sloane Kettering. I asked her how long I had to live and what I should tell my family.

"Tell them at least ten years. We are going to treat this as a chronic disease, like diabetes; like HIV," she said.

But the third antidote to my grief was the best: After the biopsy to discover what kind of a cancer I had, the surgeon came to my room and said it was good—this was breast cancer in the bone, not bone cancer. I took out my phone, the first of many times I would use Mac's picture as painkiller, as anesthetic. He looked at the phone and said,

"There are fifty new medicines for breast cancer, a pretty slow-growing disease. You had better save for his first car."

Sixteen years, I thought! And the vision took hold: me at eighty-nine, a passenger in a red convertible with the top down. I was riding next to Mac at the wheel, his tan muscular arms lustrous. And I, with a kerchief on my head, and a grin, as I faced the Pacific Coast Highway in the sun.

These were my pivotal moments to ease the grief toward acceptance. Cosmic kisses. Positive signals from the universe.

Then I started to look within for my own comfort. Or rather outward.

David Brooks in *The Second Mountain* talks about people who have joy in their faces. They are people on the Second Mountain of their lives, not those who are living for the values of the First Mountain—ambition, fame and riches.

All of these second mountain people have suffered; have spent some time "in the valley"—of crisis, illness, financial woes, loss—before they climbed this second mountain, a place which is in some way a place of giving rather than getting; of living for the good of others. But first, there is the valley between the mountains.

I was in that valley, and I wanted to know who else was in there with me.

GRIEF PART TWO

My advice is, in the beginning, let it rock you until it is done with you. And it will be over, eventually. "Be the friend of Grief, accept desolation," says Rumi. Otherwise, as psychologists say, if you put off or deny the realization until a later time, the pain may return with a double whammy.

For instance, women undergoing divorce often grieve sooner than their spouses. Some husbands may ignore the marital rupture at first. But then, say, four years later, they suffer a more profound impact.

My own experience decades ago as an abandoned wife with two very small children taught me the overpowering grief of losing a loved one. I remember thinking at the time it would have been easier had he died. This loss was so much worse than a sudden death because it was mixed with my humiliation, jealousy for the woman who stole my husband, and fear about caring for a three-year-old and a two-month-old by myself. Suddenly becoming a single parent was more of a blow than becoming a widow. It was grief on steroids. But it taught me some lessons about facing metastatic cancer.

Giving yourself time to really look at the "new normal" provides you with a contemplative space you will return to and return to profitably. You have lost a dream. Feel that shock and then realize you are in another part of your life. This part—whether you call it the valley before the second mountain, or as many philosophers say, the foyer, the passageway that will lead you to perhaps the most rewarding chapter of your life—is precious.

The deeply thoughtful space you carve out will be a lasting platform of comfort and peace that you will return to again and again. Trust me.

Meditation of some kind is a powerful healer. The Tibetan monk Phakyab Rinpoche and Sofia Stril-Rever, in *Meditation Saved My Life,* enthralled me with the story of how, through only meditation, he healed a gangrenous limb. He did this despite the urgency of western doctors to amputate or suffer death. This, as well as other books on healing, convinced me that the mind is a force which patients with terminal or chronic disease cannot ignore. It is *not* a woo-woo notion. It's a documented technique that brings many benefits, including health and long life.

I will address meditation several times as a universal antidote to unhappiness. This practice is foundational for so many respected experts in health and transformative habits. One of the desired effects is to quiet the often-disabling thoughts of grief. But I find this thoughtful exercise is also a ramp into gratitude.

I think one of the big solutions to grief is thankfulness. You may have cancer or Parkinson's, or HIV, but consider! You have the luxury of excellent health care, perhaps a satisfying job, a life well-lived in your memory, friends, hobbies you can still pursue, social engagements you enjoy, spiritual practices, the beauties of nature, your imagination still working, your spouse, children, grandchildren.

In my own life, the presence of a grandchild virtually drained away the deepest cistern of grief. It also mobilized me to find an intentional life, a purpose I could walk in—a way to help others by writing about my experience.

Once before, when I needed distraction in fighting breast cancer, I turned to what was beautiful. I found works of art in my then-fiancé's home to be a comfort during chemo, surgeries, and frequent anguish. This discovery of art's impact on my health caused me to write a book on surviving cancer and gave me the enthusiasm to share it with others in a speaking career on Art and Healing. Holding Mac had a similar effect on my body chemistry as looking at a favorite painting by Vermeer or listening to a Puccini aria.

Once before, when I needed distraction in fighting breast cancer, I turned to what was beautiful.

Find the art that gives you energy and keep it nearby. It will console you and remind you of other perspectives. More about this later.

—◦◦◦—

Others have taken the idea of things that bring comfort to an extreme. Grief might be seen as a passion for something or someone in this world that is no longer there. Is it sorrow for how the material of this world must fade? Is then hoarding a way of avoiding grief for disposing of things?

We might say that hoarders hold on in a pathological way and ignore the spirit which endures. Perhaps the hoarding heart ignores essence, life force, soul. Ken has come across hoarders often, but two stand out to me as demonstrating a kind of radical embrace of even the most expendable items, whether they have worth or not.

A man died in his apartment, and the owners called on Ken to find what they thought were some valuable pieces of art left on the premises. Ken saw a place where there were the usual "goat trails," small pathways between refuse, paper, all manner of objects, where one might position one's feet to walk from one room to another. When there is a fire in a hoarder's home, often a strange plastic sculpture will result from the heat melting saved plastic containers, and thus, these twisted pieces overrun the goat trails, making the cleanup even more horrible.

This person had a four-burner stove where he constantly cooked ramen noodles. It would seem this was his only menu. He would take the noodles out, squeeze the plastic envelope and flatten it so that it would fit neatly on a pile next to the stove. There were hundreds of these towering to the kitchen ceiling. Another, less tidy tower, was in the sunroom.

And here, also, was where the mail was stored. Piled on a ping-pong table, the unopened items reached over five feet in the air, and at least ten feet wide. Ken, in a fit of mischief, pulled out an envelope from the bottom of the pile. It was a Christmas card with a postage stamp from 1937. The date of the appraisal was a spring day in 1986.

But for me, the most intriguing, sorrowful, even scary scenario was in a house in Scarsdale, New York. A banker phoned Ken for an appraisal in this fancy Westchester neighborhood. Ken could not find the house because the address brought him to a lawn with hip-high grass. Wasn't this a house for sale? Not the client's home? A woman handling laundry answered the door and verified the address; but the banker was in the city working, so the appointment had to be cancelled.

Two more times, the banker postponed—by leaving notes on the door—because his invalid mother in the house did not want visitors. Finally, after Ken threatened to hand him an invoice for the missed appointments, the banker appeared and reluctantly showed Ken into a house full of piles of paper, books, and trash in the living room and dining room. The kitchen counter bloomed with open cans of food, dirty dishes. The backsplash behind the stove revealed an array of nails in the exposed wall where pans hung.

Tied bundles of laundry festooned the second-floor stairs.

The banker explained to Ken that he was about to eat lunch with his mother, an invalid in an upstairs bedroom. And then he disappeared. Downstairs Ken began his work: here were indeed some valuable paintings, such as one of the Duke of Wellington by Thomas Rayburn. And, along with the theme of royalty, a copy of Burke's *American Peerage* with a page open to the correct form on how to address the Queen. Apparently, the banker belonged to one of the Pilgrim families. His last name was indexed in the peerage book. There were more paintings in an upstairs bedroom.

Ken planned to return the next day.

That day, the client let him in and then left on an errand. Ken then started work on the upstairs rooms, while he listened for some sound from the room with the closed door—apparently where the mother resided. Nothing. Not a snuffle, whisper, or whoosh of electric fan, though it was summer. Where *was* the invalid, if not there? Again, the client appeared and said he would be having lunch with his mother and disappeared into the room with the closed door.

Ken got curious. He opened the only other door on the floor and saw what must have been the banker's bedroom: a mattress on the floor, a fan aimed at the mattress, and the usual detritus everywhere. But when he opened the closet, there hanging in perfect order were four Brooks Brothers suits, cleaned and pressed, all facing the same way on wooden tailor hangers, next to immaculately laundered and ironed white shirts. On the floor of the closet were spit-shined mahogany Florsheim shoes—four pair in formation, their toes facing front.

The Westchester banker had two lives—one for business and one for home. And what was behind the door where he had lunch "with mother"?

———

Sometimes, hoarding with a more positive motive is collecting to fulfill a dream. Edward from Brooklyn has garnered African art for decades. His apartment presents as a museum warehouse of 100,000 pieces: magnificent sculpture, drums, masks, furniture, ceremonial objects. All are organized throughout his large living room, dining room, right up to a tiny table where he and his partner dine. To walk, he has arranged those pathways we spoke of earlier. I have tiptoed through those tiny footpaths from the front door to his dining area, and it is a bewildering and humbling experience. Shall I trip in this ten-foot path in my size ten boots? Fall into this carved chair for mothers giving birth in Namibia?

Edward has labored for a dozen years to find an exhibit area for this remarkable collection. His is a holy mission, to offer the world his life work dedicated to the celebration of unknown but gifted African artisans.

What is heroic about this project is Edward's resilient valor. He never conveys the difficulty, the frustration, and disappointment of not finding the ideal context for his treasures.

There is no, "Poor me, I didn't get that donor to write a check."

He soldiers on, researching, reaching out, and—with passion—pitching his dream to the next potential sponsor.

Edward has no room for self-pity. For me, it's a prophetic sign he will one day win against the subject of our next chapter.

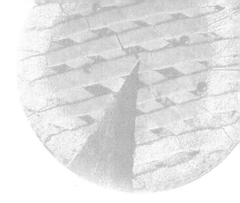

2 SELF-PITY

Always with true faith
I gave flowers to the altar.
In the hour of grief
why, why, o Lord,
why do you reward me thus?

—*Tosca,*
Aria sung by the heroine, Vissi d'Arte

Tosca's lament was mine: I was good; I had survived the tough years—single parenting my two sons. Scrimping and saving and sacrificing. I was admirable. Hey, I worked in philanthropy. I helped others give to support missions of education, health, and art—and all for those less fortunate.

PIES TO DIE FOR

So, I felt entitled to happy years in my sixties and seventies—a brilliant husband, loving and generous; beautiful home; successful kids; lively social life; travel; at last, enough money. Why *now*, cancer? This is so *unfair*.

Well, we know what happened to Tosca in the opera. She thought she deserved blanks in the firing squad's guns, but she was mistaken, and her lover died. Then, in a fit of pique and despair, Tosca threw herself off the roof.

So much for her jewels to the Virgin.

The mire of self-pity is paralyzing and is the slippery slope to depression. How to get out of it?

With self-pity, one of my antidotes is a shift in perspective, a "lift," as Mark Nepo says, that pulls us away from that slough of despond. For myself, I was always looking for company in my misery. That was my lift. I hungered to find people who suffered too.

In my grocery store, I lusted after the *National Enquirer*. Here is one of my least likable traits: sometimes I would get in the longest line in the store, so I could read for free about Julia Roberts' marital problems, Doris Day's illness, or somebody else's grotesque weight gain. Horrible delight or *schadenfreude* ensued. I am ashamed of this reflex, and it didn't help my own self-pity. It was a grotesque grimace, not a sigh of relief.

But I came across a remarkable solution related to my lowdown relish in movie star misery: change perspective. The Dali Lama talks about having compassion for others as an antidote to self-pity. And here is a guy who knows pain.

In 1959, the Chinese were trying to eradicate the Tibetan culture and people. As its leader, the Dali Lama tried hard to negotiate for and to defend his country, to bring peace between the Chinese and the Tibetans. But his efforts failed, and a devastating conflict was imminent. In the middle of the night, he had to disguise himself as a commoner and sneak away to India to save his life and stave off a massacre. For fifty years he lived in Dharamshala in exile, knowing that his people were bereft of their homeland.

Yet when the Dalai Lama speaks, bitterness and hate—the whine of Tosca—is nowhere.

Instead, he teaches that when we are in anguish, make a small shift in perspective. Really look at the suffering of another and try to understand and sympathize with that person. It will not solve your difficulty, but it will ease your pain.

. . . when we are in anguish, make a small shift in perspective.

These days, it is impossible not to find misery in the world. As of this writing, the COVID-19 pandemic gives us ample opportunities to have compassion. And there are other things too. Immigration. Wildfires. Economic woes.

I suppose I reflexively move to those close to my own condition: metastatic cancer patients. Like me, they may not be fortunate enough to have resources, skilled doctors, a loving family, yet they are also battling the same evil. I think of Kate Bowler, author of *Everything Happens for a Reason and Other Lies I've Loved*. She, too, got a surprising diagnosis of stage-four cancer, hers in her colon. But unlike me, she is thirty-five and the mother of an infant son. I am more than twice her age, and I have lived a chock-a-block full life. My boys make movies in Hollywood. I have a grandson. She has had much more chemo, surgery, and treatments causing awful side effects than I have had.

Kate Bowler melts my self-pity with an acetylene torch.

Moving away from self and self-concern is the key to this relief. I found that, at last, the habit of reading the scandal sheets in the grocery store—coupled with the philosophy of the Dali Lama and Desmond Tutu—introduced me to a more productive way of looking at other people's pain, thus bathing me in a compassion that can lessen or even banish my own self-pity.

Another strategy: whenever I like a work of art, I get curious about the artist and want to know something about their lives. Very often, the beauty of the art is in strong contrast to their lives. Vermeer's is a perfect example.

Johannes or Jan Vermeer (1632–1675) left us with a few dozen of the most treasured paintings, all scenes of interior domestic life. For example, *Girl with a Pearl Earring* is a luminous portrait so pure and light that it takes my breath away. But Vermeer died at forty-three—exhausted, depressed, and in debt. He had fifteen children. His wife believed stress, mostly over financial constraints and the fact that he couldn't paint fast enough, had ruined his health.

I think of Vermeer painting long hours in his studio with the light coming in from the left, making an effort to create such beauty in the midst of his worries. It reminds me of the humanity we all share and the gratitude we should have for the spirit of the artist, despite his troubles.

The Japanese artist Hokusai is famous for his powerful waves and his series of scenes of Mount Fuji. He moved so many times because he was focused on his work, not on housekeeping. We might call him a slob. Hokusai never cleaned his homes, but just picked up his easel and painting supplies and moved on to another apartment. Ninety-two times.

Picasso's blue period may have evolved because of a maelstrom of dejection brought on by the deaths of his sister and close friends, along with harsh poverty (Also, I read that blue, at the time, was the cheapest paint color!)

The beloved Mexican artist Frida Kahlo, remembered for her vivid self-portraits, lived a life of physical pain, but also artistic resilience. "I am not sick, I am broken. But I am happy to be alive as long as I can paint."

Paul Klee suffered from Systemic Sclerosis (scleroderma); Francisco Goya endured tinnitus and perhaps astigmatism; Georgia O'Keefe survived an intense nervous breakdown which kept her from painting for two years; Toulouse-Lautrec overcame Pycnodysostosis (prevention of bone growth resulting in very short stature).

The tormented, short-lived Van Gogh, suffered from epilepsy and perhaps a bipolar condition. He mutilated himself in his depression yet gave us glorious color and shape in his paintings.

The personal history of the artist can comfort and inspire, but there is also, as Alain de Botton and John Armstrong persuade in *Art as Therapy,* the persuasive insight of the artistic image. For example, in the Western Christian tradition, pictures of Christ's crucifixion and suffering can teach us that "pain is a part of a noble life." Art shows us the dignity of sorrow, that we are not alone in our pain, and that "sorrow is written into the contract of life."

Lightening this somber theme, Botton and Armstrong describe the therapeutic purpose of art to assist mankind in its search for "self-understanding, empathy, consolation, hope, self-acceptance and fulfillment."

One of the most interesting aspects of this theory of art therapy was, for me, the discovery of self. Learning what does and doesn't enliven you in a museum can be a healthy way to strip away numbness and uncover honest responses. A famous landscape may bore, but a wild abstract can excite. A Rembrandt may leave you cold with its picture of old age. But the visions of a Basquiat, or Keith Haring—brilliant, primitive, even graffiti-like artists—may make you say, "Hey, this is me!" Being able to express these feelings to a friend or to yourself helps you to define your needs and ultimately get what you want. The real you is within reach in these experiences, and therefore, so is aliveness.

Learning what does and doesn't enliven you in a museum can be a healthy way to strip away numbness and uncover honest responses.

Here in my approach to the inevitable sadness that accompanies a serious diagnosis, I recommend you look for the art that moves you, gives you energy. And then discover the life, the human being, behind the work. Look for the obstacles, the hardships, the poverty. Identify, if you can, with the artist's effort to make something beautiful, despite the pain. And see the possible therapeutic aspect of art. Explore the lesson about living a fuller, more authentic life in the subject matter.

And Patricia Vigderman, in *Possibility: Essays Against Despair*, does not tell us the source of her grief, but gives us her solution—writing. "[W]riting my way into and out of landscape, painting, literature, affection, sorrow and even death . . . letting different ways of being with grief, letting different ways of writing it take its measure."

Art is "a magic you can walk in and out of," she says. I found journaling and then writing, even years after my first bout with cancer, was a great comfort and then a source of satisfaction and pride that led to writing my first book, *Side Effects: The Art of Surviving Cancer*.

So, consider making art of your own! Lissa Rankin, in *Mind Over Medicine*, points out that "creativity decreases symptoms of distress and improves quality of life for women with cancer."

From the intensely personal and psychological to the global stage, art has power.

———

Art crime is the third highest crime activity in the world, after weaponry and drugs. It's no wonder when you consider that the overall art market is gigantic! According to Art Basel's *2020 Art Market Report*, even with a decline of 5 percent from the year before (perhaps due to the coronavirus), $64 billion was spent globally on art this past year. The US is responsible for 44 percent of that market, a market mostly unregulated and largely activated at art auctions. A current example of criminal activity, offered through a recent US government report on money laundering, is how Russian oligarchs use art to evade sanctions. This congressional account showed how $18 million worth of high-value art was moved through shell companies that purchased the art. The art market is an ideal playing ground for laundering money.

A story I have long found alluring about art, even if difficult to prove, comes from a truly glamorous colleague of Ken's—Nik Douglas (1944–2012). Douglas studied Eastern art, philosophy, and sexual tradition while living in the Himalayan mountains for eight years. Nik's family history could have inspired self-pity, but instead, it roused in him a swashbuckling career as an art dealer whose clients lived all over the world. He was considered one of the leading authorities of Asian art.

Nik's ancestor was, in the seventeenth century, the original, first Lord Buckingham whose son, the notorious second Lord Buckingham, became the bosom friend of Charles II, known as the "Merry Monarch." Charles loved Buckingham for lending him money, solace, and support. But Buckingham's rashness, anti-government activities, and poor soldiering got him in trouble, and he died in modest circumstances in 1687. Because of his royal connections, he was buried in Westminster Abbey. And his family was still acknowledged by the continuing British administrations.

Some recompense was made to the ancestors of Buckingham in the succeeding generations. Through the centuries, Nik's family was recognized as having a claim to a royal line. In 1890, for example, Nik's ancestor was appointed Keeper of the Stamps, a silly sounding sinecure, but with some remuneration and lots of travel expense.

In the twentieth century, Nik's father was given an ambassadorship in Cyprus, and he and his wife lived there in peace until the war broke out between the Turks and the Greeks. Nik lived there, too, but was off the island when things turned south. The British backed the Cyprians against the Turks, so Nik's father asked the English for their support because the Turks were threatening the inhabitants of Cyprus. The Brits told the couple not to worry. Soon after, the Turks invaded and slaughtered Nik's father and mother, then vandalized the home. When Nik came back, he returned to a tragic, bloody scene.

Once more, the English tried a kind of recompense. They gave Nik a choice of British holdings to live in: the Caribbean island of Anguilla or the Falklands. Nik chose Anguilla. From there, he ran a wide-ranging art dealership with warehouses in Brooklyn, Thailand, England, and elsewhere, as well as a chic boutique on the island.

Nik was one of Ken's esteemed business partners and friends. Both knew well the art market and the value of the world's prized possessions. Nik was one of the only experts I ever heard my husband defer to. In his early sixties, Nik died suddenly from a heart attack on a flight from Thailand to New York.

Whether or not we can believe Nik's history, I tell his stories because, at the very least, they magnify the artistry of his imagination, and the following story, the authority of great art—one of my beloved themes, and a consistent antidote for those of us with incurable conditions.

It was on the island of Anguilla that Nik discovered the glamorous extent of art crime, the measures to which the nefarious would use precious works to forward their schemes to gain more wealth, to eliminate enemies, and to engage in human trafficking.

Offering the most beautiful beaches in the world, Anguilla is an island for the rich who want to avoid tourism and busy, crowded resorts. The hotels are exclusive, expensive, and out of the way. So, it's not a surprise to find that on one beach there are four huge white villas facing the sea, sometimes with yachts drawn nearby. Russia owned at least one of the villas, one that Nik visited. According to his account, there were concrete lockers in the basement of the villa with carefully controlled environments for valuable art from the Renaissance, and the eighteenth, nineteenth, and twentieth centuries—all owned by various crime organizations.

When crimes were expedited, the art was transferred from one locker to another as payment. Drug transactions were apparently one of the more popular items to be paid for in this dramatic setting: a spectacular villa with a sinister basement on a Caribbean island.

Nik's story dramatizes a truth we have noted earlier—that art is the third highest illegal activity in the world. Art is a reliable currency for international crime.

As Neil Gamon observed, great art "can furnish you with armor, with knowledge, with weapons, with tools you can take back into your life to help make it better." Art has a worldwide or intimate usefulness. It can be part of your arsenal against defeatism and misery, along with meditation and a shift in perspective.

Self-pity is the younger brother of depression—a more dangerous state, a deeper dive into self-preoccupation.

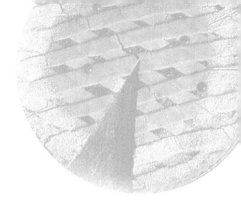

3 DEPRESSION

I tell you it has been a liberation to realize you can always find a shock of beauty or meaning in what life you have left.

—BJ Miller, physician and triple amputee

Depression can sap our energy, inject shadows in the happiest days, kill our appetites, and stain our interactions with the world. And yet, BJ Miller's quote always cheers me because it sprung out of his study of art when he became radically disabled.

As a college student, BJ was fooling around one night in a train station with his buddies. When he climbed atop a stationery locomotive, he didn't realize that it was electrified.

Thousands of bolts ran through his arm and his watch, destroying his left arm and both feet.

After many months of therapy, he went back to school and decided to take an art course that was focused on classical Greece. As he sat there in the darkness of the theatre looking at the slides, he heard his classmates respond. The sculpture of Venus—the torso of the beautiful woman with no legs and no arms—elicited a sigh of rapture from the students. They didn't notice or care that she was limbless. BJ not only identified with the statue, but he realized that you can "always find beauty of meaning in what life you have left." He went on to become a physician and a champion of hospice care. His TED talk is memorable.

Although he spoke of limbs, his words are a metaphor for the life we also have left. Depression is banished by beauty, wonder, patches of joy. We must find one of these every day. Easy to say for the one depressed! But it is a code I have tried to live by.

—⟡—

The signature quality of depression is physical inaction: not being able to get out of bed, hopelessness, unresponsiveness. I've never experienced the clinical version of depression, but I have known its dogged appearances. And bouts with it have frightened me about suicide, not being able to get out of the sadness, deepening hopelessness, and aloneness.

Oddly enough, many eloquent words have been said about depression. Famous celebrities suffer it: Winona Ryder, Dick Cavett, Lady Gaga who said, "I've suffered through depression and anxiety my entire life."

A recent TV interview captured in her own words, her radical sadness for the last two and a half years. She hired people to stay in her home with her to check her flirtations with suicide.

"I can write songs," she said, fingering the grand piano next to her, "but I can't enjoy a normal life."

There's comfort in listening to some of these famous voices speak honestly about their misery.

"Depression is rage spread thin." —Buzz Aldrin

"Depression is a wrestling with death." —Patricia Vigderman

"It is easier to say, 'My tooth is aching' than to say, 'My heart is broken.'" —C. S. Lewis

"Impossible to ever see the end. The fog is like a cage without a key." —Elizabeth Wurtzel

"Dealing with depression effectively is a mark not of weakness, but of strength." —Andrew Solomon

"Depression is not interesting to watch." —Brad Pitt

"Keep yourself busy if you want to avoid depression. For me, inactivity is the enemy." —Matt Lucas

Work on *something*. Gene Wilder said he went through periods of depression when he was idle.

YOGA

Before we get to the psychological habits that can be important antidotes to depression, I want to recommend any kind of physical movement—qi gong, physical therapy, dance, going up and down stairs, walking—on a daily basis. There is also aikido, tai chi, and other martial arts. Or try fifteen minutes a day on the trampoline, moving from side to side as you wish.

My favorite is yoga. Gentle yoga!

Thousands of years have proven that this discipline is good for the mind as well as the body. My clearly ageless instructor, Violette, constantly reminds us of what is being stimulated, opened up, comforted, and refreshed as she encourages the dozen or so seniors in our hour-plus practice every week. That's anatomically speaking.

Thousands of years have proven that this discipline is good for the mind as well as the body.

But our feelings and perspectives are also affected.

"This is time for you . . . gather your peace . . . never ask your body to do more than it can . . . open up your heart . . . open, open, aaah.

"Now bend your arms up with the elbows near your *chest.* Wrap your arms and hands and press your palms together if you can. We are going to do *the Eagle.* Ah, Carole, I know you love this one. Now put your right leg over your left and twist it a little so you are standing on your left. *Good.* You can touch your other leg down, if you need to. Keep your shoulder blades pressing down toward your *waist*. Gaze at the tips of your thumbs. Breathe.

"Now, pretend you're about to fly! Feel the muscles in your back expanding! The Eagle flies above the storm, did you know that? Release your hands and put them out like wings! Feel the air and see the clouds below! We are eagles above our stresses, great birds of strength, of freedom!"

Violette's running commentary banishes sad thoughts and reminds us of our capacity to take care of ourselves; to listen to our bodies and not worry about the perfection of the stance. For my seventy-plus years, the asanas are goals I aspire to, and that is enough.

At the end . . . it's exhilarating. Afterward, the day runs more smoothly. And I can concentrate on my second solution—a perspective on the needs of others. Which brings me to dynamic compassion.

With David Brooks and the Dalai Lama, I've been persuaded that dynamic compassion will not only distract me from illness but will also win me the years of life I crave. So, I focus on inspiring others about the healing agency of art. I use my years of college teaching, musical comedy theatrics, research skills, and even some modest success in professional speaking. With these, I build within me a diesel to move others. Perhaps it's a bargain with God: let me have the time and energy to write books, to give talks on art and healing, so I can live to ride in the red convertible with Mac Weaver.

MEDITATION

My own practice is hardly expert. I spend ten or fifteen minutes a day before I write. I listen to the Solfeggio

Frequencies on YouTube, but you may choose classical music or silence. I center my focus, close my eyes, and inhale and exhale for ten minutes. My effort is to empty my mind of things to do and settle into my heart, seeking an image of my future as healthy and happy.

Here are some simple steps I learned from neuroscientist Dr. Joe Dispenza:

- Disconnect from your world.
- Create a vision of your future self in your imagination. (healed, in remission, living with a chronic condition, but living well)
- Feel the emotions of that status; rehearse the new you. (You are a writer of three books, invited for an interview by Good Morning America, in demand for speaking engagements; selling your books like crazy.)
- Let go of your sadness, your pain, your worry. (Face a beautiful future of twenty more years of vitality.)

"The heart acts like an amplifier and goes straight to the brain," says Dispenza. When I get into my heart, I'm whole and closer to physical healing.

There's so much scientific evidence that the brain is actually changed with meditation, and one of the strongest proponents is a hero of mine. Dr. Lissa Rankin's groundbreaking book, *Mind Over Medicine: Scientific Proof That You Can Heal Yourself*, offers the most concise and dense list of the benefits of meditation I've seen, benefits not only for the mind, but also for the body. Her work, which combines science and spirituality, is one of the pillars of truth in this book, and I recommend her approach wholeheartedly.

Dr. Rankin gives us a new wellness model based on her scientific experience as a physician and as a witness to cases of spontaneous healing. She shows how thoughts, feelings, and beliefs can alter the body's physiology. Loneliness, pessimism, depression, fear, and anxiety damage the body, while intimate relationships, gratitude, meditation, sex, and authentic self-expression turn on the healing processes.

HUMOR

As Dr. Patrick Quillan says, "Laughing is good exercise. It's like jogging on the inside." Laughter is caused by humor juxtaposed to horror, and it can sometimes shake you out of the blues.

Sometimes humor comes from tragedy and even from serious international events. My husband was the chief appraiser for the Romanian government when Nicolae Ceausescu was overthrown. Ken went back and forth from the US to the city of Bucharest when the coup was happening, and he was named an authorized agent for the liberated Romanian government. Through Ken, the sale and rental were arranged for Ceausescu's 300-foot yacht. It had quarters for forty soldiers along with an array of suites, salons, and sophisticated communication technology. He was also involved in the sale of the Boeing 707 owned by the dictator.

His most vivid memory was about the execution of the President Ceausescu, his wife, and son before the firing squad. The dictator kept looking at his watch while they were arranging the firing squad. Why, asked Ken, was he looking at his timepiece? The reply came from a witness:

he was waiting for his personal coterie of guards to come in and rescue him, and his watch was connected to the leader of his guards.

The rescue never came.

It must have been a stressful atmosphere, this once-Communist society where the leader had kept strict control over women's fertility. Before the execution, there was talk of taking away all privately held farmland and putting people in agricultural camps.

You can imagine how Ken felt in this environment, even after the execution, when he heard his name announced over the loudspeaker at the airport. When he responded, he was told that two generals needed to speak to him in their offices. Ken went to the first general's office and sat across the desk from the highly decorated soldier in full uniform. The general had a briefcase in front of him and looked at Ken keenly before he unlocked the case. This was a frightening moment. When he lifted the top of the case, Ken could not see anything, only the braid on the man's hat.

"Tell me, Mr. Linsner," the general said. He grew very serious, and then pulled a pair of men's boxer shorts from the briefcase. "Do American men prefer 100 per cent cotton, or bllluuuend?"

The general wanted to start an underwear export business in America. Such entrepreneurial energy may have been a backlash against Communist rule. Next, the general's colleague buttonholed Ken with a passionate plea to help him start a Carvel Ice Cream franchise in Bucharest.

Can you imagine Ken's relief when he left those offices?

That situation reminds me of some of my favorite funny movies. Collect the titles for yourself! Here are a few of mine:

Blazing Saddles; *Neighbors: Fraternity Rising* and *Neighbors II, Sorority Rising*; *Sausage Party*; *A Fish Called Wanda*; *Elf*; *Best in Show*; *Zoolander*; *Life of Brian*.

WONDER

One of the most helpful books in my arsenal against depression is Ingrid Fetell Lee's *Joyful: The Surprising Power of Ordinary Things to Create Extraordinary Happiness*. She finds a dizzying array of elements in our everyday landscape that can bring us happiness. Analyzing our surroundings—those colors, shapes, materials, textures, activities, places, and things that give us joy and energy to live fuller lives—Lee makes an irresistible case for paying attention to opportunities for celebration, magic, play, harmony, freedom, and renewal. Depression cannot live in this array.

Reading her book is like being on a playground with three- and four-year-olds, guided by a very grown-up Einsteinian babysitter with a huge magnifying glass and an infectious and never-far-away giggle. My favorite description of joyfulness that still stays with me now, after reading the book months ago, is not one that's easily duplicated in our ordinary lives.

Reading her book is like being on a playground with three- and four-year-olds, guided by a very grown-up Einsteinian babysitter with a huge magnifying glass and an infectious and never-far-away giggle.

In Lee's chapter on "Renewal," we're taken to the cherry blossom festival in Japan. Here we find "flower blizzards" on the byways of the town; pink Kit Kat candies and special pink drinks in the convenience stores; the amazement of the residents, even as they experience an expected, cyclical, explosion of the blossoms; the pink strewn lakes and walks. I can't forget the solitary businessman walking down the street with a cherry blossom in the middle of his forehead. All these images thrilled and convinced me that we can bring joy into our lives through paying attention to the seasons, nature, art, and the wonder of our world. It is a guide to what makes life good. Read it.

TRAVEL

Even for those with mobility issues, travel can side-step depression and enhance a sense of connection with others. Train, ship, and bus journeys take you out of your head, remind you that others have sorrows greater than your own, offer transcendence in the form of new and marvelous scenes from other worlds, challenge what you expect of yourself, and best of all . . . delight.

Your first requirement: courage. Second: planning and foresight. Third: a little luck. Fourth: a travel agent who loves you and understands your pocketbook.

During my first cruise on the *Queen Mary*, I was delightedly surprised when I came out of my stateroom to see the smiling occupant of a wheelchair and his attendant coming down the gangway. Cunard builds its accommodations around these travelers—the width of hallways and the number of handicapped toilettes, etc. I found on the half dozen cruises I've experienced on Cunard and Viking that there are more than a few wheelchairs, always accompanied by energetic and optimistic caretakers. These relatives or paid attendants always seem happier than their charges, not only for obvious reasons, but also because—I believe—they're glad to share the adventure with another.

Recently, I experienced the power of travel to lift my heart, even when I was not feeling well. At the end of 2019, we took a Viking cruise to South America and an excursion to the Falkland Islands. I'd come down with bronchitis on the ship a few days before and, although I was recovering with antibiotics, I was almost ready to cancel that particular excursion because of the twenty-minute rough ride over the Falkland moor-like landscape that was required to get to the penguin rookery. But I thought I'd try the first part of the tour. So, I hiked—actually walked slowly—the half hour up a not very high hill to a most beautiful bay that looked down on a tribe of penguins. I watched their socialized swimming in the emerald water.

Most Falkland days are wet, rainy, overcast, cold, and windy. This day we were blessed with sunshine. I felt like the unexpected, gorgeous weather was a signal for me to carry on for the latter part of the adventure.

I bought a few irresistible stuffed penguins for gifts at the gift shop—also a strategic help on the bumpy journey ahead—and braved the Jeep 4X4 right out of an Indiana Jones movie with my husband and another couple.

Our driver was a blonde twenty-five-year-old Falkland native called Sally, who drove like a champion. I stuffed my penguins behind me in the small of my back—my most vulnerable metastatic spot—and held on while the jeep bucked and careened along the road. Sally was a perfect ambassador for this society of 3,400 contented inhabitants in this remote country.

Seeing the penguins close up—the real ones—was the reward for my gutsy, albeit cushioned, ride. The Magellanic animals thrust their shiny chests out and walked about together like businessmen on a mission, cared for their newborn chicks, and made me forget the cold and the wind. Mostly, they made me marvel at the contentment of the Falkland Island natives so far away from other, more conventional civilizations.

The acute simultaneity fascinated me. Some pain—my cough, the chill, the physical demand to walk uphill—was hard up against the geographical beauty of Gypsy Cove and the fascinating penguins only ten feet away, relating to each other in groups, guarding their furry young at their feet, cawing at the predator birds above.

The acute simultaneity fascinated me.

One photograph captured this paradox of death in life, or if you prefer, the juxtaposition of the weird and wonderful. You see, the Falklands still carry the wounds of war in the form of land mines that were planted on their shores during the 1982 conflict with Argentina over the provenance of these 732-plus islands. Since then, most of the mines have been removed by de-miners, experts from Zimbabwe who work in teams and wear brightly colored pajamas on the beaches to eliminate the hundreds of buried explosives.

That day we visited Gypsy Cove, we stood on the cliff overlooking the beach. Tourists are, of course, not allowed to move on these untreated lips of the ocean because of the penguins and the mines. My philosophy of vibrance in the face of terminal illness showed up in an unforgettable image, the yin and the yang. I caught both the penguins and the de-miners in the same photograph. The Magellanics are grouped at the edge of the sea. The de-miners are in their orange and yellow uniforms on the beach about fifty yards away, moving together to take their break in the hollow of the cliff. Nature at ease and a team shouting in bright emphasis of the aftermath of war's destruction were blended in one picture.

I came away from this excursion to the Falkland Islands braced with the pleasure, the grounding, and the peace of this surprising part of the world. Imperfection, limitation, great distance from other societies, incessant wind, constant inclement weather, even the marring of a beautiful nature with bombs lacing the beaches does not ruin the equanimity of the people of the Falkland Islands.

May I take their point of view into my heart and bring it out in dark times like a blessed souvenir.

Travel offers us the opposite of fake news. You are there and it is real! You smell the penguins, see their large, fuzzy offspring at their feet; look into the eyes of the woman serving you the free homemade cake in the tea house next to the ocean.

This is real, as real as the alpaca scarf you sense you must buy from them.

—◈—

It's depressing to have cancer, and then to expect to find joy in the everyday, and some sort of physical activity is essential. Travel, especially to exotic locales helps refresh the soul. But then, there's the current lockdown of the COVID-19! Here is how I have dealt with it.

When I was in school, I hated physics but was fascinated with forces, especially centrifugal and centripetal forces. People feel centrifugal force on a merry-go-round, or when a plane banks into a turn, or in the spin cycle of a washing machine, where things are pulled *outward*. Centripetal force is the opposite force necessary to keep an object moving in a curved path, such as the force of Earth's gravity on the moon, and it's directed *inward* toward the center.

In this season, I feel both—the inward and outward pull.

The global monster of this pandemic is centrifugal—outwardly spinning, overwhelming. No place on Earth seems untouched, and the canvas of disaster is huge as it flings itself to faraway places: Ecuador, Iraq, Pakistan. Places I cannot go to.

Then the opposite perspective and force intrudes, that which pulls us inward. The world reduced to our homes; our lives made smaller, more intense. Details close us in: six feet of distance, the faucet over soapy hands, masks, tiny bottles of sanitizers, the little red horns on the virus image we see on TV all the time. Our lives shrink.

I want to escape, to go anywhere from this miniaturized, closed-in world with a ravenous giant straddling it.

I miss other people but often interaction hurts. Calling businesses and services on the phone, I'm confronted with aggravated voices, cranky and tired. I suspect they're overworked because their co-workers aren't there to help them lift the tent of their labor. Their colleagues are home with small children trying to handle the stress of their dining rooms—now classrooms—and their flagging wallets. When I am infrequently out, humanity is a sea of masked strangers. No reason to smile when half our faces disappear under eyes that often project fear.

Spinning, spinning, I feel the added queasiness of my chronic illness.

All over, people and the news remind me that I'm the most vulnerable. Friends I haven't heard from in many months call and ask suspiciously, "Are you OK? Well, that's good."

My faraway sons call more frequently. I hear the weariness in their voices. "Hi Mom, how are ya doing?"

"Hey, I'm fine"

"Why don't you send Ken to the grocery store?"

"Because I just need to get out for a few minutes."

"Better be careful."

Age and my underlying condition make me a bullseye for the coronavirus.

At home daily, I'm confused, unmoored, distressed, distracted. And with all this extra time—what?—I can't seem to get anything done. The news and the internet are Towers of Babel. People trying to cheer us all up are driving me crazy, yet I can't stop reading about the free seminars for success, the quarantine jokes, the pictures of cute animals, videos of comical kids, Italians mimicking Caravaggio paintings, sorcerers who want to read my fortune, offers of $1,000 if I just fill out a questionnaire, and endless Zoom invitations.

I go to bed embarrassed at what I didn't accomplish,

My dreams offer nasty exchanges:

"Know that others are suffering too." They don't have cancer.

Realizing if I do get the virus, I'm a goner. And the danger will last for years, they say.

The vaccine will take a long time to develop. What if I get really sick, cancer sick? How dare I go to a hospital where I could get the virus?

I spin round and round, my thoughts flying off to the blue waters of our timeshare on Saint Martin where no one from New York is allowed, no one from anywhere! A closed paradise. And back to my internal worries. Our town clerk, Phil, died of the virus recently. Ken shook his hand a few weeks before.

Where are my antidotes now?

On TV, I look at the thirty-five-year-old, the sixty- and eighty-year-olds who've died from coronavirus. While my eyes fill up, the Dalai Lama's compassion kicks in.

While there are bodies in overcrowded funeral homes, Ken and I are well in our spacious home. Out here in the country, we're nowhere near the epicenter in the City. Get real. You're still very much alive. Be grateful. Have pity for others less fortunate.

The food lines everywhere sadden me. Many millions unemployed and small businesses threatened everywhere.

Change your perspective, Carole: My husband has never had more clients. Everyone is cashing in on insurance premiums for damaged art or selling their art to put food on the table. Appraising is booming. Be grateful for your blessings!

Widening the lens. You may be stuck at home, but you don't have financial issues, and there are more chances for FaceTime with Mac Weaver.

You have time to meditate, to exercise, to clean out hell holes like the garage, your four closets, Ken's library of rolled tee shirts, the laundry room . . . BUT you are missing: lunch with girlfriends, trips to the City for work or play, to Saint Anthony's in Nanuet on Sunday, dinners out, drives to Canada, to Baltimore, to Newark to, to fly to Saint Martin . . . even smiling at strangers who smile back.

The forces, inward and outward, press against me.

And yet, I still attend my Wednesday yoga class, although it's now outdoors on an enormous basketball court next to a lake, so we can put yards and yards between us.

My favorite asana is Warrior Two. Let me teach you how to do it.

Stand tall and take a step forward with one leg bent slightly before you and the other stretched out behind you. Raise your arms parallel to the floor, with the front one pointing straight ahead and the other lifted at the same level behind. Look out over your fingers. This hand is shooting light into the darkness. Or you are about to command an action. Now you aim at something high and desirable. The front arm lifts slightly. Feel the balance in your whole body.

Now say to yourself, "I AM a warrior, a female warrior, full of intensity, not aggression. I am poised for a great achievement."

Warrior Two always brings tears. Or rather, the posture fills me up. My teacher tells me that often in yoga you break barriers with your poses, and when you break the barrier, you cry.

This—Warrior Two—is the physical manifestation of delight in the body and an intention driven life. Try it!

So, I, like those the world over, fight this strange time with any physical, spiritual, or psychological weapon at hand. I blend into distressed humanity with my special burden, and sometimes I find peace.

But then there are the days when terror strikes.

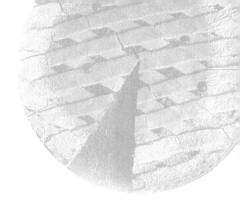

4
PANIC ATTACKS

Everybody has a plan until they get punched in the mouth.

—Mike Tyson

I woke up at 5:00 a.m. in a panic attack. I was worried about my dental problems and the connection to cancer. Did the disease jump to my mouth? Was this the beginning of the end?

My gums had been hurting for months, so at the recommendation of my dentist, I finally admitted something was really wrong.

Oral surgery was scheduled in two days. A medicine I was taking for bone health turned out to have a horrible side effect: necrosis of the teeth.

I wrapped my stocking feet around Ken's bare ones. He was sound asleep, but I could feel his hand stroke my arm. My heart was beating fast, so I started breathing deep as if I were meditating.

But sleep was impossible. I extricated myself gently and went to the closet to find a red blouse for cheer.

Calm down, I told myself. *Remember what Daddy said, "Don't worry twice." You'll start the therapy on your mouth in a few days.* At the assessment appointment, the surgeon said this was a simple procedure.

Carole in self-talk: *Handle this. Remember the panic you felt when the boys were little, and you were taking care of them alone?*

The time six-year-old James was hit by a car in the middle of our quiet suburban street? The accident was only a half block from our house. When I heard the neighbors yelling, I ran from the kitchen as if my life depended upon it.

I saw James in the middle of the street while the EMS brought out the stretcher and leaned over him, my beautiful firstborn.

"Am I going to die, Mom?" he asked. My eyes full of tears, I responded with maybe the stupidest remark I ever made, one that my sons still laugh at.

"I don't know," I mumbled.

"Mom," James, my now forty-year-old with his own four-year-old, says, "why the hell did you say that?"

My hand on the red Chinese shirt in the closet, I stopped and smiled at the memory of that panic attack that was thankfully diffused at the end of the day: James sporting a few bruises, us home from the hospital eating ice cream, and the old guy driving the big Buick that hit James, now chastened and sorry, never to be seen again on our street-loving neighborhood.

My history assures me I will survive.

Now, I was anxious but not crazy. On the porch, I did some yoga in the sunlight, especially the Eagle (my teacher said, "I am amazed you can do this difficult pose.") and then the Warrior Two. Then, to my study where I listened to the book about how optimistic recruits at the Metropolitan Life Insurance company sold 31 percent more policies than those who did not express such positivity.

I heard an ad on the radio about *Mulan,* the movie: "There is no courage without pain."

Where is your optimism, your courage, Carole?

Out in the garden to get the paper, I met my neighbor who just got a new German shepherd puppy.

"Want to see our new baby?" she invited.

"OK," I said, my heart still bruised.

But when I saw this new puppy—head leaning on my neighbor's shoulder like a newborn with his oversized paws placed gently—I melted. Here was love and nature and life.

When I finally did my ten-breath meditation in front of my computer, I felt some peace had returned.

—◦◦◦—

Living with metastatic cancer can be a hotbed of panic attacks, a never-ending river of alarm. Waiting for the results of blood tests, MRIs, and pet scans; those spikes in pain, unusual aches, most doctor visits, and hard to describe "bad days"—all these and more contain alarms that trigger intense worry and fear. Over the last four years, I've had many such moments of "rough waters" alone. I offer my personal ways of handling these ugly seas. Grab an inflatable boat and come with me.

Remember not to be necessarily optimistic or pessimistic, but one who uses "applied hope" as Thomas Friedman calls it. Blood tests and scans can change over time and don't necessarily mean the end is near. How do you feel, health-wise? Pay attention to that energy, that interior life. Not all scans are definitive. Physicians may alter medication or treatment and there may be physical changes because of that change, or the picture can improve. My own oncologist has an approach that responds to cancer markers, for example, with nimbleness: I switched from Fulvestrant to Tamoxifen in the last six months. But I had to wait between tests to find out if her decision worked. This has happened over the last four years at least three times.

Her shifts seem to be successful.

Whew.

What do you do in between the bad news and the relief? On my way to my study, after petting the eight-week-old German shepherd, I went to my Tibetan singing bowl—a big brass container a foot in diameter—and banged it with its special mallet. The resonance it triggered in my chest for a full forty seconds was soothing, and I did it again. Five hundred years before Christ, the ancient Tibetans began healing with special frequencies generated by these bowls. The dissonance of disease, these Tibetan physicians believed, melted with the alpha, delta, and theta waves into the harmony of health. Sounds crazy?

Living with metastatic cancer can be a hotbed of panic attacks that never ends.

Today, sound is being used to alleviate pain and even to cure pancreatic cancer. Today, there is increasing interest in healing vibrational frequencies. So, no Tibetan singing bowl? No problem. Listen to your favorite music.

There's no question that sound has a healing power. Oliver Sacks, the brilliant neurologist, author and researcher, created the Music Therapy Institute in New York City as a dynamic center of research on the connection. One of his most famous proofs of music's power is with Alzheimer patients. They couldn't recognize the face of their own child, but they could accompany the playing of Frank Sinatra singing "My Way" and remember every word of the lyrics. Music can thus return the Alzheimer patient to himself, even for just a little while. Sacks himself is convinced he was healed by the rhythm of a Mendelsohn symphony as he was recuperating from a complex leg injury from which, he was told, he would not walk normally again.

Don't neglect the benefits of classical, jazz, musicals, rock and roll, songs from your youth, favorite hymns, and opera. My favorite is Yo-Yo Ma playing "Soul of the Tango." Like my grandson's picture, a few bars of this changes my biochemistry for the better. I literally MUST move my body. And, with that, my heart lifts.

My last shout out to the power of music when you're panicked is to read the wonderful account of how classical guitar—well-played by a sympathetic professional artist—can awaken patients from a coma. Andrew Schulman is the only musician who is now an official member of the association of ICU physicians. He offers a spell-binding narrative in *Waking the Spirit.* Read about Mr. G who, while in a coma, was writhing in the bed, his face contorted. Andrew knew he was a retired saxophone player, so he played "Smoke Gets in Your Eyes," "All the Things You Are," and "Take the A Train." From his expression, Andrew could tell Mr. G was playing the sax in his head. And after a few hours, Mr. G. pulled through.

Or I love the scene of Elliott, a depressed British businessman and patron of the arts who was going into radiology for treatment. Andrew knew he loved the Rolling Stones, so he burst into "I Can't Get No Satisfaction," and the entire ICU "transformed into a rock concert . . . every doctor, nurse and patient began to smile and laugh . . . Soar[ing] with Elliott's exuberant energy." No wonder, the musical prescription is now, in hospitals throughout the country, part of the therapeutic plan—the trained medical musician at the ICU bedside.

Another book which is an antidote to all the monsters we fight, especially when panic strikes, is Dr. Kelly A. Turner's *New York Times* bestseller, *Radical Remission: Surviving Cancer Against All Odds.* I have it near when I feel my anxiety rising, so I can re-read some of this ten-year study of a thousand cancer patients from all over the world and how they defied a serious or even terminal diagnosis with a complete reversal.

I can re-read about Shin, dying of lung cancer in hospice, discovering the benefits of deep breathing in the early morning. On top of his condo rooftop, he noted that birds started singing forty-two minutes before sunrise. As the light came in, this—Shin's theory posits—told the birds that photosynthesis is about to happen, when the trees use carbon dioxide and emit oxygen. Shin breathed deep, and absorbed the freshest air of the day, the purest oxygen for the cancer in his lungs.

Shin also did a very weird thing: he sent love to his cancer, as if it were a sick child. Over some months, his pain decreased, and his cancer receded. Today he is living well, more than a decade after the doctors told him he had, at best, a few months to survive.

Or Susan, with pancreatic cancer, healing herself by leaving a super stressful job and using special energy movements. I guess my favorites were those who healed their spiritual and emotional wounds, those terrible stressors which make for an environment cancer thrives in. Like Joe with metastatic lung cancer, in a miserable relationship with his family, finally getting rid of the resentment and anger about his strict Catholic upbringing and his hidden homosexuality. He lives today, and happily.

So many insights emerge from these stories! Like you don't have to feel happy all the time. Emotions "should flow through you . . . not get stuck." So, when you feel panic, accept it, and then move on. The other big nuggets I've learned from Turner's successful patients are: taking control of your health, increasing positive emotions, deepening one's spiritual connection, and having strong reasons for living.

A final habit I've adopted as a response to panic is to allow some daydreaming, a kind of reverse meditation. When we focus on gaining strength and health, which looks forward to happier days, we are creating our future, according to several gurus of meditation. Daydreaming is the opposite—it can be a kind of inventory of blessings leading to appreciation.

A final habit I've adopted as a response to panic is to allow some daydreaming, a kind of reverse meditation.

Here are some of my daydreaming moments as a child in a hammock in my backyard. I am looking up at the stars and I dream of going to exotic places. I *went* to those places!! Despite my mother's sometimes violent temper, my childhood was happy with jitterbugging in the Catholic schoolyard, my uniform shaped by lots of crinolines; trips to the ocean with my family, leaving in the dark to get there early enough for a morning swim, my brother and I in the back seat with the fragrant fried chicken; college and discovering acting; graduate school and the world of poetry and Shakespeare opening to me; at twenty-two, teaching the troops in Germany and England for the University of Maryland. Ah, what adventures! All on-ramps to profound thanks.

Remembering these moments joins the heart to the brain and brings peace. And, for me, even acceptance of whatever lies ahead.

It's important to underscore this approach as one of a seventy-six-year-old who's lived a very full life. Younger people may have more stress in their lives with children and the demands of careers as they cope with a daunting diagnosis. But I still feel that remembering happy moments is a mental exercise for any age that helps us live longer.

Scientists tell us that the telomeres, those tiny caps at the ends of our chromosomes, may be one of the factors which determine longevity. The aging process, scientists speculate, is a gradual shortening of those telomeres. But we can slow down that process significantly. A recent study argues that accelerated stress shortens the telomeres. Confirmed cases of a Tibetan nun, a Pakistani woman, and a Chinese soldier prove that we can live to 100, 110, even 120 years and well beyond. When asked their secret, the common theme of these antiquarian heroes was a heart-based experience of love, compassion, calmness, and peace.

So, think of reflecting on joyous moments as a way of protecting those caps at the end of your chromosomes. Look at that list of glad times and fill your heart with thankfulness and the love you have for our dear ones.

—◦∞◦—

This story is one about a senior fellow who enjoyed life to the end.

A personal assistant married an old guy—Ken remembers him as short and stocky-—one who was rich and had lots of art. The assistant convinced her new husband to hire her sister's spouse as a security guard on their large property. The old guy put everything into a trust in his young wife's name, perhaps to avoid taxes. Unexpectedly, the younger wife dies, and the old man discovers that she has left everything in the trust not to him but to her sister. But he's allowed to live in the house until he dies.

The sister and her husband who's an ex-cop and security guard on the property, can't sell anything because they can't pay the taxes. The old guy fires the husband as a security guard, and the couple are broke!

The old guy continues to live in the house and even leads them on by having dinner with them occasionally, seeming to offer a solution to their stuck finances. But he does nothing.

Finally, several years later he is found face down in his pool from a heart attack. During the ensuing estate appraisal, Ken finds women's bathing suits in the changing room next to the pool. After careful examination, the sister of the old man's wife identified the swimwear as owned by women other than her sister or herself. The old man apparently had a healthy romantic life before he expired.

Life is amazing, unpredictable. Consider the surprises of this story: the younger wife dies before her husband who was twenty-five years older; the old man might have expected all of his possessions to come to him. After all, he was a pretty good husband, right? But no, the wife pulled a fast one and left all to her sister! The old man had a place to stay for as long as he lived, and he was surrounded by his art, even though it really didn't belong to him! The sister and her husband owned it all but couldn't sell it. They were house and art poor! Then, another surprise!!

The old man's heart gives out, maybe because of his romantic involvements in the pool. The sister and her husband had to sell everything to pay taxes. The house became part of a local college. Life! Be ready for it all!

One thing we can say about the old guy: he didn't elect to be lonely. Our next chapter confronts that demon that hangs around so many of us, sick or well. Some say it's an epidemic of our time.

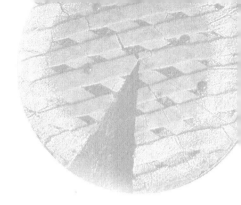

5 BATTLING LONELINESS

The opposite of loneliness is love.

—Dr. Vivek Murthy, 19th US Surgeon General

D r. Vivek Murthy, in his nationwide inquiry into the health of Americans, found that 20 percent of adults suffer from loneliness. Not just an occasional sad feeling, but a condition that damages their lives. As told by Kate Bowler on her podcast, lonely people have less productive workdays, for example. And surprisingly, greater than diabetes, obesity, or smoking more than fifteen cigarettes a day, loneliness shortens lives.

AARP: The Magazine published an article in the December 2019 issue called "Is There a Cure for Loneliness?"

Through seventy studies that followed a total of 3.4 million people for an average of seven years, the article confirmed that loneliness adversely impacts lifespan. Each of three groups—those who were socially isolated from other people; those who described themselves as very lonely; and those who lived alone—all faced the same increased risk of an early death: 32 percent; 29 percent; and 26 percent respectively. What's noteworthy is that physical health or lack of it was not a factor. "Whether or not you are healthy, those who are more socially connected live longer," the article stated.

Yes, you say, cancer and other serious illnesses also shorten lives! But put in the context of our culture where technology can connect us but also keep us from genuine interactions; where the roots of families have been spread out across the nation and the world; and where it's harder and harder to make connections that last and nourish each other; having a life-threatening disease will surely worsen the sense of isolation. Especially in the current context of the COVID-19 pandemic.

To be sure, the cancer community does offer online remedies, including message boards on such rich websites as SurvivingBreastCancer.org. These are especially welcome for those with mobility issues.

You can join a support group based in a hospital or reach out to your oncologist who most likely has access to a social worker (I've found this to be true at Memorial Sloan Kettering). Also, there are numerous cancer centers listed online by region, and women's centers are also good sources of regular group meetings, lectures, fund-raisers, and other events, virtual or in person.

WORK ON A PROJECT THAT HELPS OTHERS

Become a fund-raiser, you say? Help raise money for a cause? Why would I do that if I'm not feeling well? Take it from an old fund-raiser—doing so can take your mind off feeling lousy and really boost your popularity if you're feeling left out. For the past thirty years, I've worked in the vineyards of philanthropy—raising funds for hospitals, colleges, arts organizations, and start-up non-profits. I found it to be an amazing engine for the greater good, but also a monumental way to bring satisfaction to see people working together for a common cause. Fund-raising for missions I believed in kept me healthy and happy for decades, despite a stressful life as a single parent.

Philanthropy—writing grants and proposals; face to face asks; persuasive communication in all genres; creating events—these are some of the methods used to raise money from alumni, patients, sponsors, and other donors. I still do this as a part-time senior consultant. I enjoy being in the marketplace rather than the classroom, and I'm grateful for what I learned.

I respect philanthropy's deeply American impulse to give as the way this country developed its original institutions, shaping bright cities and towns out of the wilderness with churches, orphanages, hospitals, schools, colleges, museums, concert halls, and public buildings of all kinds. Alexis De Tocqueville (1805–1859), a French diplomat who visited the new world in the nineteenth century, was astonished at the way Americans pulled together to make life better for themselves and especially for others. So quickly, so naturally. He watched them meet on the street to discuss the next project with enthusiasm and effectiveness. There was happiness in this work.

And this national spirit survives. You can share in it.

I'm not necessarily suggesting that you take a job with a nonprofit, but I urge you to consider giving your time to help others. You can even do phone calls from your home. Volunteering for a cause you believe in—cancer or HIV research; a children's project; your local hospital, synagogue, or church—can do wonders for your frame of mind and even your social life.

I'm not necessarily suggesting that you take a job with a nonprofit, but I urge you to consider giving your time to help others.

As Dr. Murthy and David Brooks have said, we have become a deeply individualistic society, which is one of the structural pillars of our greatness but also our loneliness. The civic, community connection still thrives in parts of our country, but so many of us have lost that original sense of *Who am I in relation to others? What can we build together?*

We are each other's solution.

As Dr. Murthy says, "Loneliness may be the disease, but we are the medicine." Aim for a broader perspective than that of your problem, disease, diagnosis. You are *not* your wound.

In a related approach, Dr. Silvestri's book *A Wider Lens: How to See Your Life Differently*, teaches us to broaden our perspective, to expand our frame, in order to embrace pieces of ourselves and those pieces related to us so that, by being aware of the bigger picture, we can be more whole, become stronger, and deal with difficulty more effectively.

Dr. Silvestri, using various tools such as systemic psychotherapy, mindfulness, homeopathy, coherent breathing, and Aikido (a martial art based on peace and harmony), teaches us that *context* is more important than *content*, and *connections* rather than *fragmentation*. As a patient with a serious diagnosis, I see my whole life—past, future, and present—as a rich and precious experience, one to be continuously grateful for. I'm not meant to dwell on the pain and fears of cancer, but to embrace the totality of life, of *my* life.

Mindfulness, being in the present moment, equanimity, open mindedness, and reasonable positivity—these are the gifts of seeing with the wider lens. Dr. Silvestri's book is really helpful, whatever difficulty, whatever problem you are facing.

EXPAND THE FRAME

Let's consider how my husband Ken has learned how to expand the frame of his own talents.

In addition to his appraisal prowess, Ken is also a master conservator, a repairer of art objects. I've seen this first-hand. Once he was given the challenge of restoring a large oil painting of a naked woman that had a jagged three-to four-inch hole through the middle of it. It looked like someone had, in anger, smashed a fist through the image of her naked back. Ken worked on the painting in his lab a good portion of the day. The following morning, I peeked into his workspace and saw the smooth flesh of the woman.

The hole was gone! Somehow, he had rewoven the gash in the canvas and then, with his skill at inpainting, returned the glowing pinkish orange of the skin to the image. Even up close, the surface looked perfect.

This talent is an extension of a fault of Ken's, a deficiency transformed into a magnificent capacity. Ken went to medical school intending to become a thoracic surgeon. With superb grades, he was on track, but as an intern on hospital rounds, he found that he could not treat patients. They exhausted him. The sickness of others depleted his energy, despite his mastery of textbook knowledge and techniques. Being an empath prevented him from practicing as a physician.

Later in life when he turned to appraising and examined paintings, sculpture, ceramics, etc., his medical skills re-emerged. At the heart of his training was passion for chemistry—the Materials of Art was a course he developed and taught at New York University. And surgery—subtle hand movements guided by keen observation and anatomical mastery—was his special strength. So, he applied his love of nature's intricacy, of returning wholeness from damage, of *healing* to a new arena. He widened the frame of his focus on medicine to the restoration of damaged works of art.

A delightful client of his mirrored this ability in an almost comic pivot. This physician purchased a minimalist painting. Usually, minimalist art of the 1990s has a white background with very little interruption of the surface, but sometimes with a rich texture. The doctor decided to put the painting in his examining room. It was, after all, created by a famous Polish artist and the doctor was from Poland. When his landlord decided to paint the offices, the doctor left the painting on the wall. The painters didn't recognize the large white object as a work of art, and they painted over it—white on white.

So, the doctor called Ken to ask him to repair the painting. Ken told him the process to restore would be costly and time consuming but said he would do it. After some thought, the physician replied.

"Ahh, no. Let's keep it this way. The painters were also Polish, so I can still say the painting was done by my countrymen."

He "expanded the frame" and continued to value the painting as one created by Polish hands.

SUPPORT GROUPS ARE THE ANSWER FOR SOME

I'm not a regular joiner of groups. Metavivor (for those with metastatic breast cancer) is a website you would think I would belong to, but I would prefer not to, even though I think they're correct in saying that 25 percent of women with breast cancer find that their cancer has metastasized. I am in that percentage. Breast cancer research is terribly remiss in not devoting more to this too-frequent aftermath of ordinary breast cancer. And I applaud Metavivor's advocacy for this kind of research.

But as I explored the site, I was discouraged when I came upon their posting that this one had died. That one had died. And they talked about how long they'd lived with the diagnosis. This depressed me, so I moved away.

To me, *SurvivingBreastCancer.org* is a more attractive online support group. "From day one" is their tagline, and they focus on the many ways breast cancer patients can improve health, beauty, and attitude. I spoke for them once in the City, and then became part of their speakers' group. I have done enjoyable webinars on "Art and Healing: How the Power of Sound Can Make Us Better;" "How to Get It Done: Your First Shitty Draft," and "Pies to Die for: Some Ways to Get out of the Dumps with Metastatic Cancer."

To me, SurvivingBreastCancer.org is a more attractive online support group.

Embrace your strengths, and don't remind yourself of the fatality at bay.

For me, most cancer support groups depress me. I prefer to come across cancer survivors and their stories of heroic triumph. I like the fresh impact of individual stories like Olivia Newton John's (more about her later) and that of Valerie Harper who famously said after the return of her cancer in 2013, "Don't go to the funeral before the day of the funeral." She died in August of 2019 at age 80, living well beyond her doctors' predictions.

I encourage, instead, meetups or interest groups. The real answer for me to combat loneliness has been the National Speakers Association/New York Chapter. Life affirming, energizing, and inspiring, these once-a-month meetings in the City (now, virtual) have been worth the annual membership fee (about $800 for about eight meetings). NSA/NYC has expanded the frame by encouraging my blended loves of college teaching and acting into a burgeoning, rewarding speaking business. How I enjoy these successful professional speakers—about one hundred strong—who share their messages of hope and their secrets for building careers! Wow, no wonder their annual conference is called "Influence." These stars move hearts and minds the world over. This is my community.

Life-long learning is one of the key reasons I embrace the National Speakers Association. I gain wisdom from the topics of the speakers, from the arcs of their careers, their mistakes and triumphs. I never feel lonely amongst them.

On the other hand, crooks expose themselves to the self-imposed loneliness of prison for the lure of crimes' rewards.

As mentioned earlier, big money can be made in the world of art crime. In insurance fraud, however, the sums may be smaller, but the criminal mind still works overtime. Here's an example of cheating that is first preceded by what the insurance companies call "a trial run"—a toe in the water, so to speak—before the bigger plunge.

—◦◦◦—

Trainer Claims are insurance claims that the insured makes to test what the insurance company will handle—or if you will, fall for. One such trainer claim was from an attorney who called to say he was afraid to leave his wife's jewelry at home while he took an extended business trip. So, he put the gems in his office, ostensibly to be safe. Sure enough, there was a theft while he was away. When he put in the claim, the company duly paid $20,000 for the stolen jewelry.

Thus, a trainer claim.

Now comes the real event.

During a storm, a tree fell on this same gentleman's house. The damage within was substantial. But what was worse was the robbery that ensued. The thieves had defecated in his crystal glasses and took an ax to his antique table. They shit on his Japanese futon. They peed on his tapestries from Tibet and smashed what he said was a priceless porcelain elephant. Horror and destruction.

The insurance company said they would pay to replace the locks on the doors, but they needed receipts for the other items.

The man sent in a bill for the futon: $4,000.

The crystal elephant: $3,500.

The antique desk from Rome was tagged as $26,000.

The insurance company called in Ken to investigate these claims. Ken first took the receipt for the elephant. It was from A to Z Imports in New York City. Ken travelled to the store and asked the clerk if this was their receipt.

"Oh yes," he said.

"Will you show me the crystal elephant that costs $3,500?"

The clerk showed him a six-inch swizzle stick with a tiny elephant on the top.

"Oh, no," said Ken. "I'm looking for something much more substantial. About eighteen inches."

The clerk looked puzzled.

"This is the only elephant we have."

He showed Ken the display in the front case. The price tag? $3.50.

Ken looked at the receipt again and saw that the decimal point had been turned into a comma, and two zeros were added. So much for the crystal elephant.

The antique Italian table was more difficult. The receipt indicated a charge of $26,000 from a store in Rome, and while the description of the table was there in typescript, it was difficult to read. Squinting, but determined, Ken found the phone number of the store and called.

"Do you sell fine antique furniture, like a special nineteenth century hand-carved desk?"

"No," said the Italian store owner. "We are a jewelry store. We sell only fine jewelry."

Looking hard at the receipt, Ken shrewdly observed that two documents had been blended by two typewriters: one was European, the other American. The Italian one had the letter I with a pointed top; the American one had a flat seraph top. The attorney had used the main part of the receipt from the jewelry store and doctored the description and the price.

The $4,000 Japanese futon was even easier to scuttle. Ken found the store that was selling futon covers for $40. With the same forging hand, the attorney added two more zeros and presented the receipt as real.

The insurance company, spurred by Ken's revelations, invited the man to come to their office to finalize the last payment to cover his losses. He arrived with his wife who was wearing a beautiful diamond tennis bracelet.

"What a lovely bracelet," said the welcoming agent. "I suppose this was one of the pieces that was replaced by us when it was stolen from your husband's office. Looks great on you!"

"Stolen?" replied the wife. "Oh no. I never take this off. My dad gave it to me when I graduated from college. Since then, I wear it all the time."

The agent then turned to the attorney to ask the question. Suddenly, the attorney put his hands together to say *time out*.

He asked to speak to the insurers in private, away from his wife. He realized that they knew what he'd done.

"I'll give you back the money, and we can forget about it."

And that's what he did. He gave back everything, including Ken's fee for investigating the claims. Even so, the insurance company called the New York Office of Insurance Fraud, and he went to jail for three years and was disbarred as an attorney.

LONELINESS WITH REVENGE?

Ken was called to an estate appraisal on the upper west side in New York City. The apartment house had a concierge, and Ken was expecting an elegant setting. The woman who died had an estate worth $20 million. Let's call her Jane. She was alone most of her life, the single beneficiary of her father who had left her $10 million. All Ken knew about her was that she'd built up her father's legacy and passed away. She was in her late sixties, a widow of about three years.

The living room was the first shock. It was drab with a thin navy rug and what looked like IKEA furniture—simple Scandinavian lines but made in flimsy wood, somewhat battered, and not much of it. The only newer piece in the room was a blue couch, traditional in style, a Macy's product perhaps. There was a single chest in front of the couch, a simple bench across from the seating area, one easy chair, and a two-shelf unit upon which a forty-inch TV from Costco sat. The dining room was even more spare with no curtains on the windows and a simple artificial flower arrangement on the mock-mahogany dining table.

Jane had lived alone in this setting for thirty-five years and apparently didn't often see her extended family, including siblings. Her one connection to her family was a young nephew. She had allowed him to live with her while he was enrolled in law school, and she seemed to develop an affection for him over the four years they were under the same roof—with or without him paying rent. We aren't sure. All went well, until he met a girl at school and announced his marriage and departure from the home. When he came back from Geneva for his honeymoon, he gave an expensive Swiss watch to his hostess. Ken found it during the appraisal, tucked under miscellaneous items at the bottom of a closet.

Tossing that watch onto the floor of the closet may have been a metaphoric gesture—of spite? Of rejection? Or was it a preface for her next move after her nephew got married? At age sixty-five, she chose the best friend of her deceased father—a ninety-four-year-old invalid in a wheelchair—as her husband. They lived together for a few years before his passing. Another legacy she collected: her husband sold his business and left everything to her. Jane managed to cultivate her legacy with outstanding acumen, growing $10 million to $20 million over several decades.

When she died, she left all $20 million to the Red Cross, the Metropolitan Opera Fund, and the ASPCA.

Nothing was bequeathed to her family.

When you crave closeness with others, don't forget your extended family, especially those who live far away. FaceTime, social media, Skype, and Zoom are all ways you can connect. And connection relieves loneliness.

Perhaps I'm reading into Jane's life, but it would seem she had very little taste or talent for intimacy. As for the law-breaking attorney who made false insurance claims, it's interesting, isn't it, that his wife knew nothing of her husband's crooked schemes—a failure of loving familiarity that ushered in a career punishment for the attorney.

A healthy intimacy is one of the foundations for a healthy life.

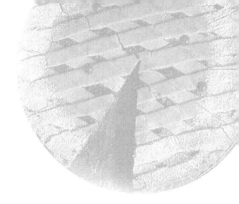

6
INTIMACY PROBLEMS

Ah my deare angry Lord,
Since thou dost love, yet strike;
Cast down, yet help afford;
Sure I will do the like.
I will complain, yet praise;
I will bewail, approve;
And all my sour-sweet days
I will lament and love.

—George Herbert, 1593–1633

I love to lie in bed when Ken gets up before dawn to go to work. He is very quiet in the bathroom next to our bed, so I doze while he performs his morning rituals, only the sound of the water running under my very shallow sleep. I keep my eyes closed and wait for my favorite part. He is fully dressed now and goes to the long credenza parallel to the bottom of the bed. Here is a ceremony that never alters: putting on his watch and jewelry and counting some money in a certain drawer. It is still very dark, so I can only hear the tiny sounds of gold against gold, of leather against wood, the soft rustle of arm into jacket and hand putting paper into pocket. Somehow manly sounds, a kind of song to a sturdy vanity; a salute to completion and readiness for the day. I love the consistency of a personal ritual and the sense of crisp tidiness. I wait to hear the last gesture: closing the credenza drawer, and he turns. I know I will get a kiss at the end. Cool and slightly perfumed skin and mouth.

Awake, so awake is my love. And then he is gone.

In case you missed it, I really do love my husband. His brilliance, humor, manliness, kindness; his superb smile, and easy laughter, excellent taste and sense of style. The way he has stayed with me despite my faults, my fears, my terrifying health crises.

But these days, I miss our romantic life.

Since my diagnosis, I think that my husband doesn't find me as sexually attractive as he used to. At least our sex life is not what it was. I researched "sex and cancer," even "sex and breast cancer," and found a few promising stories of thirty-somethings describing their acrobatic adjustments with mastectomy, chemotherapy. Their husbands seemed eager and happy to adjust. But this was not an answer for me.

But these days, I miss our romantic life.

When I asked Ken about our intimacy, he said that his reluctance had nothing to do with my cancer, but only his own health concerns (an irregular heartbeat; sleep apnea that he's trying to correct with a CPAP machine—not a sexy contraption in bed. When I pressed him, he brought up an argument we had months before . . . I turned him off with my rage "like your mother.")

Or is he afraid that he would be making love to one who is dying?

In our seventies, perhaps I'm unrealistic to ignore the multiple factors that reduce the sex drive in my partner. After all, he is loving to me in so many ways . . .

Sometimes, we need a lesson in contrast.

———

When I went to the Apple Store to take a class with my new MacBook Air (a gift from Ken), I passed by the store window of Victoria's Secret and stopped to look at the display. Could it be that simple? Become like the leg in the black-patterned stocking and bejeweled high heels—the picture I'd discovered under Ken's bathroom rug one day? He'd clearly been masturbating to this image. Was this a signal for me to get a little more pornographic in the bedroom? I'd been hurt and a little shocked, but I took some action. Sort of.

So, I wandered into the store for the first time in twenty years and met a saleswoman, let's call her Dawn, who understood immediately that I wanted to be sexy without going broke. We connected so quickly that we were soon confiding about our partners. She lived with a guy who was abusive and exploitive, expecting her to work seven days a week so that he could have health insurance. Yet he constantly berated her, descended into depressions and ate dinner over the sink with his back to her, then flew into tantrums over small habits like the way she cleaned dishes. But he was constantly eager for sex and was very good at satisfying her.

I told her about my ideal husband: kind, funny, hard-working, orderly, fascinating, generous, excellent cook, but not terribly interested in me sexually it would seem. Dawn and I were two pieces of an unhappy puzzle. I have what she desperately longs for; she has what I need, or what I think I need.

Touching is an essential part of loving. Dr. Rankin marks "a healthy sex life" as an important ingredient in healing. But there are other options beside sex. Take a look at BJ Miller's frank article, "Is There Sex Life with a Terminal Disease?"

So, I went to my friend, Sheila Pearl, dubbed the "Love Doctor of the Hudson Valley," and I complained.

Touching is an essential part of loving.

"I know about failure to thrive in babies. How about in senior citizens? I need to be touched too! One of the reasons I go to physical therapy is because of the fifteen-minute massage at the end!"

Sheila suggested that I try to connect with Ken any way I could.

"Take opportunities to stroke, give short spontaneous neck massages, hug, sit side-by-side to watch TV, offer little kisses, plan occasions and events together. Talking, cooking, playing golf together, dining, exercising, and walking can also offer the pleasures of intimacy without sex. Sometimes these are the connections that generate warmth and the closeness that we all crave.

"Thoughts are things," assured Sheila. "Always convey loving thoughts, and he will respond."

I've found this to be helpful, if not the total solution. Taking responsibility for my affectionate gestures really does have an effect on Ken's demonstrative ways. These days I'm content and grateful with the lovemaking we share in our daily and nightly rituals, our rich and marvelous relationship, with or without sex.

W. H. Auden may have the final say about uneven relationships. It speaks to me these days as the ultimate understanding of my own commitment to love:

> How should we like it were the stars to burn
> With a passion for us we could not return?
> If equal affection cannot be,
> Let the more loving one be me?

With others also—am I imagining this? They seem cooler. Even close friends, some of whom seemed to have drifted away, or else their spontaneity and responsiveness has waned. Are they seeing me as not long for this world? Maybe they don't want to be reminded of my disease. They seem to handle me gingerly. I get the sense they're reluctant to be honest, to disagree.

What works for me is a combination of acceptance and technology. With friends, welcome their tenderness and care if they express it. Even their worry. For those close or far, I offer them an update by e-mail every six months or so that gives them a general picture of my medical status along with a generous dollop of news from my extraordinary life (e.g., scan is stable, although blood markers are a little heightened; medication is changed slightly. But feeling great! Let me tell you a bit about my new project . . . a play about appraisal adventures for Penguin Rep. The director is interested. Face time with grandson in Hollywood . . .)

But I can't help it: the cooling of intimacy reminds me of death. How, the hospice nurse said, dying patients shouldn't be touched so much by their families and friends. The touching disturbs the patient because they're between two worlds, and the warm hand of a son or friend wrenches them back to the living when they may be easing into transition. She explained that the reason some people pass when their family is gone from the hospital or the room where they lie is because the dying want to be alone as they merge into the next world. It's easier on them. The cooling of intimacy is perhaps a natural reminder, and it should be respected for its signal of the next world. When I think about this, I think about what I will leave behind.

LEGACIES

Those closest to me sometimes remind me of my passing, even if I try to avoid the thought. But when I do think about it, I'm reminded of what I will leave behind. Legacy, after all, shaped my professional life for years as a fund-raiser.

I directed planned giving at the college where I worked, cultivating aging alumni to remember their alma mater in their estate plans. I learned that a legacy can be gifts of companies, insurance, real estate, time-shares, all kinds of art, and pets. But then there are psychological legacies not articulated in documents for the living.

The story of Subash stands out in this regard. The father of one of Ken's colleagues was a successful purveyor of stolen temple items in the 1930s in India. He would sell the items on the world market for hefty prices. Into the woods he would send henchmen, dark operatives called the *Daku*, to steal statues and pieces of sacred buildings. One day, the *Daku* demanded more money. The father refused. Outraged, the thieves kidnapped his seven-year-old son and demanded payment. When the father still did not pay, they sent him the ear of his son in a beautiful box. The mother exploded. The father sent the ransom. Subash was finally retrieved, forever scarred.

Later he became a wealthy owner of a shop on Madison Avenue where rare art objects from India, China, and Tibet are sold. Ken often dealt with Subash in the appraisal business. He knew him so well that he spent time in the shop, even wandering around the building where Subash kept his store of goods. One day, Ken was in the basement and met Kumar, an associate and talented restorer. Kumar was dressed for Madison Avenue, but he was working on a wooden horse with tools and paint brushes. Familiar, Ken approached him thinking that the workmanship was about repairing the paint:

"Interesting," said Ken. "What are you doing with this piece?"

Kumar, "Well . . ."

"What historical period is this, anyway?" Ken asked. He was looking at what seemed to be an antiquity.

Sheepishly, Kumar replied, "If you stop me now, it will be eighteenth century. If you let me work an hour or so, it will be seventeenth or even fifteenth century."

Forgery—or art crime-—in Subash's basement was a vignette that signaled both the curse and great opportunity of the appraising profession. It also foretold the fate of Subash.

I met him in person one day in his dimly lit, sumptuous shop. Inside, everything indicated *only the rich shop here.* There were niches with a saffron glow. Not many pieces visible. Then Subash himself emerged—or rather materialized in the dusky light. Elegant and handsome, he wore a gorgeous silk Armani suit and tie. He did not smile but fixed his brown eyes on me with a kindly intent. I tried so hard not to look at his ear, but when he turned after asking me my purpose, I could see the mutilated shell scar around the hole that was his ear. Funny, how that flap of flesh—when it disappeared—accentuated what it should announce: the cavity ushering in music, seductive words, the hushing of mothers, the click of a Mercedes' car door. Subash could still hear but without the curved embrace, that wonderful subtlety of flesh.

The store made me feel my roots as a steamfitter's daughter, not the wife of an esteemed appraiser who knew the owner well. I left quickly, welcoming the heat of the pavement so much more direct than the rarified air of the gallery.

Years passed and I heard nothing about Subash. Then one Sunday, Ken suddenly shouted above an article he was reading in the *New York Times*. It was a photo of Subash in handcuffs. He, too, had become a thief of temple objects and was caught by import police.

Now he languishes in an Indian jail, where the only comforts of furnishings and even adequate food are those brought by family or kindly outsiders.

From the father to the son, some legacies are dark and deeply cut.

———

The story of Nipsy Russell—comedian, dancer, actor, poet—shows what other surprises can occur in legacies. If you look him up, you'll see a charismatic star of mostly game shows from the 1960s through the 1990s. Shows like The Dating Game and Hollywood Squares. He was famous as a creator of poems like:

What is the secret of eternal youth?
The answer is easily told;
All you gotta do if you wanna look young
Is hang out with people who are old.

And this:

Spanking a child to get him to learn
Is something I cannot defend,
How can you knock any sense in his head
When you're whacking him on the wrong end?

Julius "Nipsy" lived in the Henry Hudson Hotel in downtown New York City. There were over a thousand rooms in the building but only a dozen were economy size, the size Nipsy chose to live in for many years.

His space was about five hundred square feet with a bathroom at one end. He built shelves for storage on one wall and put in a single bed attached to another wall, allowing him as much floor space as possible.

The impression was of a tiny apartment.

Nipsy never had luggage when he travelled, and he travelled a good deal. He liked to condense his suits and costumes in vacuum bags—the ones where you suck out all the air after packing, so it flattens out everything inside—and he would put his clothes in these bags, pair shoes with them and then FedEx them to his next performance location.

Nipsy made good money doing movies, television, and personal appearances. He had two girlfriends: Gloria, an African American, and Terry, Caucasian. Gloria was a beautiful nightclub singer he met at the Bristol Hotel in Geneva, Switzerland. He took her to Berlin, got her a job, and they became lovers. Then he put up Gloria in her own New York apartment that he bought for her.

He met Terry on a cruise ship and hired her as his official photographer. She followed him around to various gigs, supplying Nipsy with pictures for celebrity magazines and newspapers.

We know all this because Gloria hired Ken as the estate appraiser for Nipsy when he grew ill. Ken started to take inventory in his hotel home even before Nipsy died. Nipsy was in the hospital for some time with stomach cancer, and both girlfriends would come visit him there. There he was in Lennox Hill hospital, a girlfriend on each side of the bed.

Gloria was especially pushy.

"Nipsy, I'm not getting any younger. Why don't we call in Reverend Martin and tie the knot right here?"

"Glo, honey, you don't want a wedding in no hospital room," he responded. "I'll get over this in a few days, you'll see. Then we can have a real party in that restaurant on sixty-third street we like so much."

"But Nipsy, the doctor says . . ."

"Don't pay attention to him. I've got nine lives! Besides, why are you pushing to get hitched, honey? You know you're the major player in my will."

"I want to be your wife," she answered, "not a player on paper for a dead man! I've been your woman for the past ten years! I have my pride!"

Nipsy didn't think he was going to die, so he continued to assure her that they had time.

After Nipsy's demise in 2005 at eighty-seven, Ken recommended that Gloria go to Nipsy's relatives in North Carolina to make sure they were all right with his legacy plans. He didn't want anyone to contest the will, especially without a marriage to assure the bequest.

Gloria traveled there immediately, and told his aunt and uncle directly, "Nipsy left everything to me in his will. We were like husband and wife, sort of." She stumbled here, remembering the girlfriends. "I just don't want you to feel that I'm a gold-digger . . .".

"Never you mind, Gloria," they answered. "He took real good care of us over the years. Generous checks at Christmas, and he even paid off the mortgage on this house. We don't expect anything more."

Indeed, Nipsy was worth at least a million dollars. There was money to spread around.

In fact, when Gloria wanted Ken to do the appraisal work at Nipsy's, she sent a limo to pick him up.

Nipsy liked to invest in bearer bonds, and he put his cash in these dangerous instruments. They were somewhat risky because anyone who held the physical papers could cash them; in this case $200,000. And when Nipsy died, there was a major brou-ha-ha from his main squeeze.

"Ken, I am so upset," Gloria said. "Where are the bearer bonds? The will said they were coming to me, but I looked everywhere . . . and they're gone."

"Wow," Ken said. "And whoever has the bonds, has the money. No one needs to identify themselves to cash them. Let me try to find them."

But Ken's s search for the bonds was futile. He also noticed that another valuable item was gone: an expensive Hasselblad camera that had sat on one of the shelves.

Why was the camera gone? No one had a key to the apartment except Gloria and Nipsy's agent. Gloria called the police.

Under questioning, Terry—the other girlfriend—broke down and confessed her anguish at not being included in the will. She'd gotten the key from the agent, slipped into the apartment, stole the camera, and grabbed the bearer bonds with the intention of dividing up the spoils.

Both the agent and Terry were ultimately prosecuted and served time. Gloria retrieved most of the bearer bonds.

—◦◦◦—

A caretaker of a ninety-four-year-old man called and asked Ken if she could sell her charge a piece of art for a million dollars. She said she had a purse with a famous painting on it. But she couldn't think of the name of the artist who painted it.

Ken asked her to send a digital picture and told her that it looked like it was Van Gogh.

Her charge told her that he would pay her a million dollars for the purse.

"Where did you get the purse and who did the painting?" Ken asked.

She told Ken that *she* had painted the purse. "How much could I get for it?" she persisted.

Ken said, "The art market is based on what people will pay."

"Would you put that in writing?" she asked.

"No," Ken said, exasperated with the woman. Ken would not risk his reputation for someone determined to trick a vulnerable buyer. And yet, his expertise has often rescued others who found themselves in financial disaster.

Ken was friendly with a couple who'd gone through a divorce from their previous mates. Earlier, he'd been helpful in advising one of these husbands, Chip, the son of an owner of a famous department store chain, regarding the value of the art that was divided between himself and his soon-to-be ex-wife. They had acquired the collection from the estate of a deceased friend. Neither Chip nor his wife at the time had an idea of the country of origin. They just assumed that most of the items were from Asia.

They'd contacted an auctioneer who offered to give them $12,000 for the collection, which was comprised of a few Western pieces in addition to what the couple assumed were mostly Chinese pieces.

As an afterthought, Chip contacted Ken for advice. Ken soon found that the first two vases were Korean from the twelfth century, and later at a major auction house, they fetched $42,000 and $36,000 respectively. The balance of the collection was sold in excess of $100,000.

The division of the property for the divorce was a happy conclusion.

So, it was natural that Chip would call on Ken again when he found himself in another financial pickle with his new partner, Vanessa.

Chip was in serious money woes when the family trust set up by his ancestors was suddenly terminated, effectively cutting off his income for an uncertain length of time, an income that fueled his wealthy lifestyle. He was accustomed to a steady stream of income from investments, but now he faced a long wait time to reinstate funds when the trust would be dissolved among heirs. How to survive?

He called on Ken to help him liquidate some items he hoped could be auctioned as soon as possible.

Ken picked up the phone and heard the strained voice of Vanessa on the other end. "How are you, Vannie? I haven't heard from you and Chip for a while."

"Oh Ken, we are in deep trouble," she said. "We're down to our last couple of hundred bucks. And the furnace is making weird noises. It's freezing here, and the lawyers don't have good news about our income."

"Let me change my schedule around, and I'll get there as soon as I can," Ken said.

Unfortunately, the timing was terrible. Chip and Vannie—a dynamic, athletic, and philanthropic blonde—were living in a small house in a country village with their belongings in an adjacent garage. It was Christmastime. As Ken drove up, snow fell outside the huge wooden doors, and the light from the overhead lamp inside cast a soft glow on the furniture. Boxes and artwork were stacked against the walls.

Ken got out of the car and hugged Vanessa, who wore a scarf wrapped around her head. It reminded him of the Russian waif Ninotchka. And there was Chip, his face red with the cold, holding a tarnished silver candelabra in one hand and sorting through an old trunk with the other. Ken was used to seeing his friend in more opulent settings—at fancy country clubs, on yachts, and inside the pastel mansions of Connecticut. The couple welcomed him warmly as the snowflakes accumulated on the driveway. Ken went to work.

"Ken, I'm so grateful you're here," Chip said. "I hope you can find a few things we can sell," he laughed, "so we can put food on the table. Am I in a Dickens novel?" he quipped.

Vanessa held up a fake palm tree with silver leaves and a silky green bark. "Hey Ken, we have two of these! They're from the El Morocco Night Club. When it was closing, we asked the owner if we could buy the trees for our foyer. Cute, heh?" She smiled ruefully.

Ken nodded, frowned; "Hmm," he said, stroking the bark and snapping a picture. "Maybe a stage prop?" He walked deeper into the barn.

"What about this sleigh?" asked Chip.

"That could be useful for a department store holiday scene," Ken said.

"And the snow leopard hide?" asked Vanessa.

The three bundled against the cold, sifting through their belongings to find something they could transform into their grocery fund for the next few months. Ken took notes and thought about comparable items on the market, so he could price the items. And fast.

In the next two weeks, he put a number of their items into a well-known auction house. The snow leopard hide brought $15,000 alone.

A year later, Chip and Vanessa had weathered the storm, reestablished their income through careful investments, and spent a lot of time on their redeemed sailboat, *Caribbean Girl*.

On land for a few months, they invited us to their home. Chip let me drive his elegant antique car, a dark green Bentley from 1938. What a treat! It took all my strength to keep the big lumbering vehicle on course. But I loved the gravitas of the heavy turning mechanism. Handling it was serious business, but I was rewarded when other drivers in this swanky beach town nodded and saluted respectfully. Maneuvering that beautiful machine through town, I learned what it felt like to be truly, truly rich. But I also remembered that snowy Christmas when these members of the 1 percent tasted the fear of encroaching hunger.

Chip and Vanessa changed after this crisis. Like me, they'd had a wonderful life that was seemingly destroyed by the fiscal end of their easy income. I, too, was comfortable after one bout of cancer and didn't expect the surprise of metastatic return. We had both confronted a valley of sorrow.

But they turned to other resources to get through, the treasure they each had accumulated over the years. And not only did that give them some time before the trust was distributed, but it also gave them a different perspective on life. They became happier and more generous on their Second Mountain, where David Brooks says life moves "from self-centered to other centered . . . where we embrace a life of interdependence, not independence. And we surrender to a life of commitment."

Vanessa's philanthropic instincts bloomed, and the couple became a beacon of charity in their community. The last time I saw her, she was wearing a gown and getting ready for another gala to raise funds to support research into breast cancer cures.

As for me, after the initial grief, I found that through the psychological and spiritual practices outlined in this book, I am in the happiest, most satisfying part of my life. Facing the limitation of my days on earth, I stand on this second mountain, and offer this book to you—perhaps while you are living in your valley—with love.

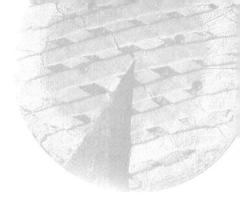

7 INFORMATION OVERLOAD

*Getting information off the Internet is like
taking a drink from a fire hydrant.*

—Mitchell Kapor

The point of this chapter is to encourage you to be
careful about using the internet to discover the
newest treatments for cancer or other serious health
conditions. I'm basing my recommendations on my own
mistakes, missteps, and discoveries.

I constantly browse the internet for answers myself,
but I've learned to use my doctors, published books,
some publications by cancer centers, and other patients
to corroborate herbs, remedies, and medications which

claim to cure. Perhaps the essential hunt should not be for a cure. Some day we may find a cure for cancer, but in the meantime, I'm seeking healing—a total experience of mind, body, and spirit.

In this chapter, I've done less complaining about sites that I believe have a commercial motive and, instead, offer my favorite authors and websites which, over time, have proven to be legitimate, enlightening, and helpful. Above all, I favor the integrative medical approach. That is, doctors who blend the conventional with the homeopathic or naturopathic approach. As you know, the triad of chemo, radiation, and surgery is the standard protocol for cancer, but more and more conventional doctors are turning to nutrition, epigenetics, and alternative methods to treat patients.

Dr. Brownstein, a popular integrative doctor, told a recent webinar audience about preventing COVID-19 with an important insight. In the early part of the epidemic, he was called by New York doctors who worked in the ICU.

"What do we do? These patients are dying!" they implored.

When Brownstein suggested a vitamin C intravenous drip, they doctors asked, "Give that to them in the ICU?"

"No," said the good doctor. "Give it to them earlier—in the ER!"

What's encouraging is the effort the doctors made to reach out for homeopathic methods, even as the physicians were fighting on the front lines with conventional medicine. I believe that the best doctors and younger physicians move between these two camps of healing.

Lately I attended a Zoom webinar about prostate cancer. In the initial survey, the attendees were asked where they got their health information. The response, published on the screen, showed that 95 percent of the forty attendees said, "The internet."

This didn't surprise me, but it did alarm me that we're in an age when vetting information is too often outweighed by the overwhelming amount of information that bombards us. When I Googled "cures for cancer," there were 2,930,000 sites. The amount of information becomes a blur if you're wondering whether or not to recommend chemotherapy to your sister-in-law, despite the fact that she weighs seventy-two pounds and has a type of cancer that normally doesn't respond well to chemo. Or if your grandson should get a flu shot.

It is not just the enormous overload of information, but also the *dis*information that's out there that's troubling. Too often, I've been lured by a newsletter that promised a radical remedy to my lousy sleep patterns and found that I wasted twenty minutes on a video and was then directed to buy a product that costs $40—and it may or may not work!

It's probably useless to suggest that you avoid surfing the internet. But I think it *is* important to try to avoid information overload by choosing sites that honor the following design:

- It's simple.
- The information is relevant.
- The website is clear.
- It provides supporting information.
- It offers balanced information.
- It's easy for the user to take action.

Watch out for fake news. Find the trustworthy sites by being skeptical about unverifiable information; obscure news outlets (ever heard of the publication?); grammatical errors (fake news writers tend to stumble); or a suspicious domain name. The best site I've found for this kind of guidance is https://wordtothewise.com/2019/01/whats-a-suspicious-domain/

Always be a little skeptical about what you find on the web.

Watch out for fake news.

Here are some sources of truth that I highly recommend:

- TheTruthAboutCancer.org

Ty Bolinger and his wife, Charlene, are real champions for successful alternative treatments for cancer. I recommend his 2016 book, *The Truth About Cancer: A Global Quest*, as a corrective to all wrong information overload. Their website and their community are also impressively current and encouraging for anyone with a cancer diagnosis.

For example, their last conference in Anaheim, California, October 11-13, 2019, offered a host of sessions from physicians, scientists, and political leaders from all over the world. I'm only including a sampling here of two of the forty-one presentations. These are cutting edge, exciting developments in allopathic, alternative, homeopathic, and integrative medicine.

1. Dr. Patrick Quillin, "12 Keys to a Healthier Cancer Patient"

   The twelve keys include: 1) finding the underlying cause; 2) understanding the underlying solution; 3) the importance of attitude and mind; 4) genetics and epigenetics; 5) energy alignment; 6) exercise; 7) microbiome; 8) detoxification; 9) nutrition food and supplements; 10) why nutrition works; 11) change the underlying cause; 12) rational cancer treatment.

   A rich overview of how current integrative oncologists are using, instead of the standard protocol of surgery, chemotherapy and radiation, the premise that the body can heal itself through natural means, especially the right mindset, diet, exercise, lifestyle changes, and the "doctor within you."

   Dr. Quillan is an eloquent proponent of "writing yourself a prescription for happiness" and the abundant science behind how we can reduce our chances of getting cancer.

2. Dr. Leigh Erin Connealy, "The Cancer Revolution"

   Presenting the essential elements of her 2018 book, *The Cancer Revolution: A Groundbreaking Program to Reverse and Prevent Cancer,* Dr. Connealy outlines her tests, treatments, and therapies she's used with over 45,000 patients at her Cancer Center for Healing in Irvine, California. Dr. Connealy believes that the new medicine, Integrative Medicine, can and does prevent—and even cure—all types of cancer, but only an individualized approach to each patient will work.

She explains and recommends many different types of tests, even those that can predict cancer within a decade of manifesting a tumor, so that patients can change their lifestyle and nutrition for optimum health. She offers hope for the future of oncology through many different types of therapy, from infrared saunas and other light treatments, mistletoe, oral health interventions, and precision-based immunotherapy using CRISPR technology. A worthy presentation at the end of this two-day global conference on cancer.

- Chris Wark is a young man who had cancer in his twenties and cured himself. He's very approachable and passionate about his mission to help others. He focuses on nutritional pathways, herbs, and supplements. You'll find Chris's book listed in Appendix 4 Reading List. He often gives webinars in which you can ask questions. Once you're on his e-mail list, he'll send you invitations to his webinars.
- Kate Bowler's, *Everything Happens* podcast is vibrant, upbeat, and inspiring. I love her prayers and her guests! Kate is a pancreatic cancer thriver. She's in her late thirties with a happy marriage, a young child, and a big teaching job. She chooses relevant topics, not all cancer-centered, but philosophically, she is very in tune with the themes of this book. Highly recommended. See https://katebowler.com/podcasts/
- Jeff Neurman is another witty commentator who speaks with wry wisdom of his own cancer experience. Amusing, articulate, and honest! Here's a guy I could be friends

with. Read his account of people who annoyingly give you advice about how to treat your disease when you've just gone through months of chemotherapy. Visit his website at https://ItsInMyBlood.blog/

- Here are some well-known sites for cancer information and support:

> The National Cancer Institute
> American Cancer Society
> Cancer.net (voice of the world's cancer physicians and oncology professionals)
> CancerCare.org (especially counselling, support groups, and financial services)
> The Cancer Therapy Adviser

If you do find an interesting theory about cures, ask one of your doctors. I usually ask my brainy doctor, Dr. Berkowitz. Just don't forget that there's safety in numbers. Ask more than one physician their opinion. These days, in contrast to more than ten years ago when I was first treated for breast cancer, I'm finding more and more integrative medicine manifested in cancer centers. Acupuncture, massage, and yoga, for example, are offered by Memorial Sloan Kettering cancer departments. Integrative medicine is blessed by the physicians, although it's not covered by my insurance.

And today there are more ways of treating the often-terrible side effects of chemotherapy. Thirteen years ago, when I underwent chemo, it was not called "an infusion," which makes it sound like a cup of exotic tea. Today, chemo at NYU Langone Health is offered in single, private curtained areas where you can enjoy reflexology while the IV is administered.

I highly recommend becoming enlightened about what are called alternative or holistic treatments. They range from nutrition and IV treatments to heat, light, and sound programs, from essential oils and herbal teas to combinations of special diets, a range of supplements, and detoxification strategies. There are remarkable options to the standard protocol, and they are worth exploring.

There is a LOT happening in cancer research and cancer cures. Inform yourself and keep asking questions. Find those you trust, like a reputable integrative oncologist or an expert in cancer care who is willing to talk to you.

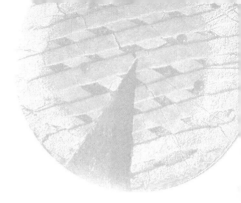

8
DOCTORS

A single arrow is easily broken but not ten in a bundle.

—Japanese Proverb

*I*f you can't find a brilliant integrative oncologist or a clinic for your ailment that makes your heart lift, aim for a blend of traditional and alternative healers. See them as a team.

But, most of all, heed the advice of Lissa Rankin, author of *Mind over Medicine: Scientific Proof that You Can Heal Yourself.* She calls your "inner pilot light" the foundation stone upon which everything else is built—including work, mental health, creativity, spirituality, and the capstone (but the most fragile) physical health. The inner pilot light is the "inner knowing, the healing wisdom of your body and soul that knows what's true for you and guides you, in your own unique way, back to better health." This is an excellent guide to selecting the physicians and healers for your team.

After my diagnosis, the first doctor I met at Memorial Sloane Kettering was a research star. Dr. L. seemed remote. When she assured me that cancer care would likely give me a decade more of life, I felt coldly comforted. Life with a chronic condition seemed reasonable, even hopeful. Immediately, she recommended a new immunotherapy drug called IBRANCE®. I was encouraged.

But as it turned out, she was a scientist with hardly a bedside manner, or was she just too busy? I started taking the drug and had an appalling reaction. After two weeks, death seemed more desirable than continuing this immunotherapy. Her office in the City was difficult to reach by the phone, and the actual trip into downtown New York with traffic and parking was extremely stressful. Only her nursing assistant would speak to me the many times I reached out to Dr. L., as I leaned over the phone—nauseated, exhausted, and scared.

After almost three weeks, despite my family's urging to stick with IBRANCE®, I stopped taking the drug.

I needed a different doctor.

The hospital placed me with Dr. D., nearer to my home. Dr. D. was the head of oncology at the Harrison Branch of Sloan Kettering—about thirty minutes by highway from my home. She is the metaphoric heart of my healing team. Dr. D is a deeply sympathetic physician with more than a little Chinese culture flavoring her western medical approach.

She, in other words, believes in the power of the mind and spirit to heal. Always greeting me with a hug, a smile, and an appreciative look at my appearance, this slender, pretty woman with shoulder-length hair, enters the windowless exam room like a flash of sunlight accompanied by a spring breeze. She makes it known—and I don't care if it is a strategic white lie—that I'm her favorite patient. When the news of the PET scan or blood test is not very good, she lets her nurse practitioners go over the report with me first. They are excellent and kind, her handmaids. Sometimes I cry with them, knowing the doctor will come in the room eventually and fix things.

She . . . believes in the power of the mind and spirit to heal.

"Let them give her the hard truth," I surmise her thinking.

It is as if she doesn't want to taint our intimate joy together. When she finally comes into the room to address the shadow on the liver or the spot on the lung, there's no direct mention of these scary developments—only what she intends to do. In the most recent case, she changed my medication. It has been working well to keep me alive these three years—her adjustments in my treatments, which she calls "tricking the cancer."

But I know what really keeps me vital are her words at the end of the session, the food she offers for my spirit.

"Tell your brother you will have many more birthdays."

Or, when she sees my face fall. "You are meant to be here for a long time. Your books, your speaking work that inspires others, fuels that."

Once she told me my picture is on her refrigerator at home.

How can I fail her?

Dr. Keith B. is quite the complement to Dr. D. Intellectual, cool, a lively scientist and researcher, experienced with alternative approaches to cancer, he's a model of the effective integrative physician. The rumor is that he only takes hopeless or very serious cases. His practice would be overrun if he were not selective.

Oddly enough, the patients in his office look healthy and happy. I am one of them! Are we hiding hopelessness? Or is he the generator of this positive atmosphere?

There's no warm and fuzzy bedside manner; just a pleasant assurance of a whip-smart physician loving what he does. Dr. B brings comfort through his wide-ranging knowledge of new medicines, supplements that seem to be working, new therapies, and—interestingly—the history of those outliers who treat cancer successfully without chemo or radiation. He's always tapping on his computer when I meet with him, looking up my new treatment from Dr. D. or exploring some substance I heard about on The Truth About Cancer.

Dr. B. is my brainy partner. He never contradicts Dr. D., and he always makes me feel like I'm on the right track, or he gently suggests another way (e.g., more vitamin D3 when he sees my blood test.) He also guided me when I came across a foundation that works on healing cancer naturally. This is the Beljanski Foundation, a European organization that offers education on world-famous treatments. They developed an herbal supplement I take and which, I think, has helped bring down my cancer markers. Dr. B basically vetted the directors of the foundation and encouraged me to make contact with the Beljanski group. I'm very happy that I did.

Practitioner Y is a functional medicine expert, and, as they used to say about the army, she knows cancer patients travel on our stomachs. Ms. Y was a surgical nurse for ten years before she studied the wide-ranging power of the gut. She monitors my blood, my body mass, and especially my diet. Y has educated me on the demons that provide a hotbed of growth for my cancer: sugar, gluten, glycemia, acidic foods. I buy my vitamins and minerals under her surveillance. Mostly, she's given me a code to live by, one that I don't always follow, but I wince if I don't obey. Y is my conscience. When I take a bite of the chocolate donut, I see the image of her scowling face in the icing.

M is my Japanese acupuncture practitioner. When she inserts the needles, she uses thirty of them, instead of the usual ten. M is a holistic healer who addresses the mind, body, and spirit in a lyrical and deeply expert manner. Essential oils, mindsets, behavioral panaceas, even special ceremonies for the new moons are part of her retinue of holistic health approaches. After her treatments, I feel both peaceful and energized. I call her the soul of my healing team.

In addition to these four, I depend upon my pharmacist who runs a country drug store just down the street from my house. Over the last four years, his charges for my medicines are incredibly low. Larry gives Big Horrible Pharma a good name. I also have a pain doctor who monitors my blood every three or four months to make sure the gabapentin I take three times a day is working properly. And, finally, I have a superb dentist, Dr. H, who keeps my teeth and gums healthy—an important dimension of a strong immune system threatened by cancer.

Together, these are my guides with different lanterns, like those of Dante's Virgil through the Inferno, or other Saints through the *Purgatorio*. Heaven is the cure, and we have not reached that yet. So far, I need all of them with their varied strengths and visions of how to get there, or at least, how to keep travelling as we move onward with prayers and their distinctive beacons of light.

Speaking of travelling through exotic realms, I must tell you the story about Ken's work with art that was looted from the Nazis. Perhaps this contains some of the most dramatic characters, one with great meaning for my thoughts on legacy. For another, the plot has significance regarding our decisions about doctors. As our healers have everything to do with recouping our health in the midst of a frightening diagnosis so, also, experts can recover stolen art over generations, creating a thread that joins us to the past and may even define the tapestry of our heart's desires.

Much has been told about the recovery of stolen art from the Nazis in their lust for valuable paintings during World War II. Ken was hired by one family in the States—I am calling them the Miller family—who wanted to retrieve certain paintings their family owned and which they believed were in a small-town museum in Germany. They didn't want to actually re-possess the paintings, but they wanted proof of their existence, so they could apply to the German government for monetary restitution. For that recompense, they needed an official appraisal of the works. Thus, Ken would have to see the paintings in person.

Ken wrote to the museum and asked about the paintings, but the curator refused to answer and would not return his calls. So, he decided to travel to the German museum. Even with a nasty cold and a nastier museum manager, Ken saw that all but one of the paintings were on display. During his research, he found out they were worth millions.

There was another reason the family hired Ken. Earlier they had engaged an attorney to find out about the paintings before and during the war. The attorney, digging through the voluminous files of death certificates, wills, and other business transactions kept lovingly by German bureaucrats, found a will leaving a woman—we shall call her Susan somehow related to the American family with German origins a modest share in the estate, seemingly a small amount, decades earlier, but the attorney—named George Merkel in my account—suspected it was now quite a handsome sum.

He then did an illegal, and unethical act. He tracked down the woman and called her, Susan Pearl, offering a business deal—a reward he thought she should give him for finding the will and her legacy.

"Hello, this is George Merkel, Esquire. You don't know me, but I'm doing some legal work on behalf of the Miller Family in Pittsburgh."

"The Miller family?" Susan said. "They are distant cousins, I think. Yes, what do you want?"

"My news for you—uh, it's really a gift!" he said. "In my work in the German archives, I discovered a bequest named for you, Susan Pearl, by a deceased member of the Nikoff family."

"Nikoff?" she asked. "Didn't they own a publishing house years ago?"

"Yes. The Nazis took it over in the late 1930s."

"What does that have to do with me? What bequest?" she asked.

"I'm calling to tell you that you're probably a very rich woman," Merkel said. He then signed her up to give him a percentage of her inheritance. When the Miller family found out what Merkel had done, they sued him.

And here's how the fortune found its way to Susan Pearl: In the 1920s, Noah Nikoff owned a publishing house that specialized in producing art books devoted to Jewish artists living in Germany. He and his wife, Ruth, also collected art, mostly expressionist paintings by German artists. They worked together to create a thriving business until in 1934, when Noah died. Ruth continued to run the publishing house, but when the Nazis climbed to power, she decided to send her two daughters to Canada. When she chose to sell the publishing house and follow them, the Nazis stepped in and told her she must first pay a tax before she could leave. Ruth paid the tax and tried to leave again the following year.

But the Germans repossessed her passport and forbade her to leave without an additional payment that she could not afford. This plunged Ruth into despair. She went home and put her head in the oven and died. It was 1939.

The Nazis immediately took over the publishing business. They also discovered the considerable collection of paintings that were included in the will and confiscated them.

Later, George S., a wealthy manufacturer of ball bearings during the war became interested in the Nikoff art. Since ball bearings were used to produce weapons, the Germans probably paid him for the crucial hardware through barter—the paintings in the Nikoff collection, those found by Ken in the small, private museum.

These art works would not be returned to the family. But the German restitution law would still pay the American Miller family for those stolen art works.

Meanwhile, Ruth Nikoff's will, it is surmised, said that the housekeeper should receive a percentage of the estate. She embraced the housekeeper and child in her legacy. Ruth may have been aware of the dangers of staying in Germany while the Reich governed, and with her death, some resources would be needed by the housekeeper and her child to leave Germany when they could.

We don't know what happened to the housekeeper and her child. But we do know that the will George Merkel discovered stated that part of the Nikoff legacy would go to the housekeeper, who then left her legacy to her daughter. And she left it to Susan Pearl.

Susan Pearl was not aware of this bequest until Merkel uncovered the documents.

Ken worked with the Miller family to take Merkel to court. Perhaps the judge was baffled by the details of the tangled wills and decided not to prosecute Merkel. At least this defendant had done his part in helping to find the paintings.

Ken's appraisal of the paintings looted by the Nazis was $4.5 million. We don't know what the family received in recompense, much less the portion that was awarded to Susan Pearl, because the German decision regarding the restitution remains in a sealed document.

That court case, with the recovery of art stolen during the Third Reich as a fascinating backdrop, demonstrates the importance of legacy even unto the third generation; the prevalence of Nazi greed and, at the same time, Ruth Nikoff's humanity. An acute simultaneity.

The inference of Ruth Nikoff's kindness is a bejeweled strain in the story of this bequest. Ruth's compassion for another woman and her child portrays the regained art with an aura beyond the art itself and the award to the family and Susan Pearl.

The travails of our ancestors, their strength—sometimes in the face of horrific circumstances—their passions, and their decisions surely shape our dispositions and our heart choices. I believe that our authenticity has roots in understanding our forebears. The more we know of our relatives, the more we confront their mystery, the more we come face to face with complexity. Why did they marry *that* one? Have too many children? Why did they leave their mates and marry another, cross the ocean to a strange land, endure miserable work lives, die young, or last into their nineties despite drunkenness, poverty, and ill health? But the inscrutable motives and the distant details of their lives mark us, I believe, in flashes of unexplained preferences and even the fleeting conditions of our souls. Are the answers whispered in our genes, or are our brains and hearts marked in some way by our ancestral history?

Brooding about those who have gone before is a privileged and accessible habit these days with Ancestry.com and other genealogical sites. I believe this cultural trend honors our own lives by looking back in a mirror at those who were indispensable players.

—⁓◈⁓—

I offer this foray into my own quest for authenticity. It is based on hearthside research, lap-hugging hearsay, fragments heard as my mother gossiped with my aunts, while I, a curious ten-year old, listened in the other room. But valid genetic information or not, it speaks to my artist heart, as you shall see.

My own great grandmother on my mother's side is a dim figure sketched by a few facts offered by my mother, the youngest of nine children, the last living repository of family lore. Her father, John Dubiel, hated the French because his apparently-French mother had abandoned him and his twin sister, sending them to America when they were quite young—eight or nine years old—and alone.

The name Dubiel sounds French, (pronounced *doo-byel*), yet it is actually Swiss (there's a town in Switzerland called *Biel* and *du* means from). His mother may have come from this French-speaking area, or from France itself, specifically Alsace-Lorraine. John, my mother remembered, despised his French heritage, sometimes muttering curses against Alsace in his cups of homemade beer.

John preferred the Polish part of his inheritance. His father was a general in Napoleon's army. He was much older than John's mother. Comically, John tried to change his name to Dubielski, but the judge threw out the request. If my grandfather's face held any hints in the one photograph that I have of him, his mother had magnificent green eyes, an aquiline nose, and a strikingly seductive smile.

Still quite young, not even in his teens, John tracked his mother down in Biloxi, Mississippi, where there's a French-speaking culture. Here the details end in a theatrical scene of the young John looking up a flight of stairs in a house next to the river where his mother lived. There, she refused to acknowledge him as her own.

John and his sister grew up as semi-orphans, raised by perhaps an aunt or cousin. Some shred of detail lingers from my mother's musings—the house with the stairs was a brothel, his mother a prostitute in the Mississippi port.

Now that I'm facing the end of my own life, I can't help but wonder about her. I note my tendency to be a Francophile. I can understand more of that language than speak it. I feel at home with French people and places.

---

*Now that I'm facing the end of my own life,
I can't help but wonder about her.*

I'm preoccupied with outrageous, rebellious women, especially those who abandon their children. My own experience was that my husband left me for a younger woman, me at forty with two very small boys, she in her late twenties, working in the same advertising industry as my husband. Some aspect of my great grandmother's fate—only in reverse—has marked my own life. While raising my sons as a working single parent, I was often depressed at the thought of those jam-packed years and thought of myself as a distracted, worry-ridden, bad mother.

I yearn to know the truth. To touch her name or her son John's name on the plaque there on Ellis Island. What was she thinking? Feeling? What did she wear? Did she travel alone?

Perhaps her mystery is one of the reasons I write—to flush out and finish the story of the passionate woman who made radical decisions, my great-grandmother who may be hovering above my fingers as I weave this rich tapestry.

Doctors, our team of healers, led by our inner pilot light, guide us forward. With the flashlight of our ancestral story, however bright or wide its glow, we see more clearly who we are and perhaps what our legacy is and might be. But however sunny our path, darkness can interrupt with the shadow called pain.

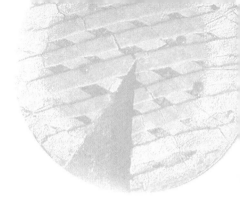

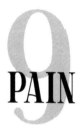

PAIN

Pain—has an element of Blank—
It cannot recollect
When it begun—or if there were
A time when it was not—

—Emily Dickinson

I almost didn't write this chapter because I believe that, while pain is a universal condition, handling it is a private and most personal decision. I hope it will give you, if not a remedy, a pathway to courage, compassion, and understanding.

Pain is still the greatest challenge of medical science. Research tells us that the body has no specific area where the reception of pain resides. We know the main receptors are in the brain—not that the brain itself hurts. "Unless the brain tells us, there is no pain," says Bill Bryson in *The Body: A Guide for Occupants*. With new technology and magnetic resonance imaging (MRI) we can watch how the brain reacts in real time, but we still don't know exactly how or why. So many mysteries stymie us. For example, phantom limb pain occurs in the part of the body that's been amputated. As Brysen so elegantly states, pain is "a burglar alarm that won't turn off, even after the theft has occurred." It can torment a soldier who's lost a leg for a lifetime.

Pain is still the greatest challenge of medical science.

The McGill Pain Index, a rating scale developed in 1971, allows individuals to communicate the quality and intensity of pain they're experiencing to their doctors. It rates pain from complex regional pain syndrome—some of the most severe pain that starts at 40—to toothache pain at 20. The McGill chart puts cancer at 28, just above migraine and under fibromyalgia.

While this index may be helpful for some patients, it doesn't take into account all the variations. For example, initially, the pain in my back was closer to 35 and it was keen, relentless. More recently, it's varied from a toothache to probably 30, depending on my physical movements. The McGill language for description of pain is also unsatisfactory: what is the difference between "miserable" and "horrible" or "aggravating." Probably the one to ten scale used in hospital rooms and accompanied by smiling or frowning faces works clumsily but best. It's what I use most frequently to describe my experience to my doctors.

The two major types of pain give us an insight into the pain's longevity and also perhaps, its origin.

Acute pain is good pain because it has a purpose—it signals that the body rejects the hurt, but that healing is beginning, and the body part will get well again. Chronic pain, however, stays with us, often as a useless reminder. Cancer *chronic pain* is the worst because it normally settles in well after the first attack of the disease when pain should have announced its arrival. I, for example, did not feel pain in my back until years after the metastasis started there. Chronic pain is a broken part of the system, the highest signal of futility. Chronic pain, like cancer cells growing, shows that the nerve system has gone haywire, continuing on and on, when it should have stopped.

Forty percent of people in America have chronic pain, including those of us with stage four cancer. And we can blame either the original cancer or the subsequent treatment of chemotherapy or radiation for this hamster wheel of pain.

Before I tell you about my own wrestle with pain management, I want to take a brief, deep dive into the history of pain treatment. Melanie Thernstrom's *The Pain Chronicles*—an extraordinary study that weaves together enormous research, science, literature, riveting prose, and her own story—gave me a healthy outrage, wide-eyed incredulity, and then a powerful dose of compassion followed by a fragile comfort for all of us in pain and those who hope to understand us.

This chapter could be more meaningful if I shared with you a little of Thernstrom's saga, especially about what our ancestors experienced. We are wildly fortunate in comparison. Pain may be "blank" in terms of when it begins, according to Emily Dickinson, but the stories of those who've suffered before us can act as an analgesic for our own struggles.

We may not be able to eradicate our suffering, but compared to Fanny Burney (1752-1840), we can bow our heads in grateful relief from what she endured. For Burney's mastectomy, performed by Napoleon's surgeon in 1811, she was given only a few sips of a wine cordial for the excruciating pain. Fanny's family could afford two mattresses for the ordeal in addition to seven men to hold her down. Fanny's own account a year later, even 200 years in the past and read by a culture steeped in horror films, curdles the blood.

Through a cambric handkerchief thrown across her eyes, she could see the glitter of polished steel. So, she writes, I "began a scream that lasted unintermittingly during the whole time of the incision—& I almost marvel that it rings not in my Ears still! so excruciating was the agony." She lived another twenty-nine years.

In 1811, Abigail Adams Smith (1765–1813), daughter of American legends John and Abigail Adams, also underwent a mastectomy without anesthesia to remove a cancerous breast. She lived only two years after the operation. (Ironically, Fanny Burney's breast was likely not cancerous; Abigail's was, and thus the reason for her shortened life.)

Some Renaissance paintings show breasts that may, indeed, have been cancerous. And, what about the ones we don't know about—countless women in convents who weren't allowed to show a doctor a diseased breast, and thus suffered for decades before they died?

Why do the surgery at all? Breast cancer without surgery gave not only pain, but also a great open wound and a stench that turned sufferers into introverts, much less patients willing to show their breasts to healers with knives.

Appalling to me is the history of anesthesia—why wasn't it used earlier when nitrous oxide and ether were both available?

The Pain Chronicles asserts that the main reason was the strong culture among surgeons who insisted that pain was necessary, beneficial, and even sanctioned by God. Crying was a sign of health. The unconscious patient was considered in a temporary death during the procedure and this state had to be avoided. Surgery had an intractable prejudice against pain relief.

It was 1846 before the first anesthetic was used for surgery. 1846! Imagine the agonized humanity before that date: wounded soldiers with diseased limbs, those with tumors or stomach ailments—all that required the merciless scalpel. On October 16, 1846, Dr. William T.G. Morton convinced his fellow doctors that ether was convenient and helpful, thus dividing medical history in two forever. (For a description of pain during my first bout with cancer in 2007, see *Side Effects: The Art of Surviving Cancer.*)

As for me, in early 2016, after the disaster of IBRANCE® with my first oncologist, I was prescribed several different kinds of opioids because of back pain; oxycodone and fentanyl were the most notable. And they had terrible side effects: incessant nausea, diarrhea, debilitating fatigue, and insomnia. I just couldn't handle the impact on my system. The pain was mitigated, but at what cost? This experiment lasted three months, and I spent most of my time praying for sleep or hanging out in the bathroom.

Finally, after my incessant complaints, my pain doctor gave me a much milder medication called gabapentin, which I've used daily for the last four years with, as far as my pain doctor and my team have seen, few or no side effects. Three hundred milligrams, three times a day surely must have or will have some effect on my system, or God help me, my memory.

When I bring up the subject with my various doctors (I'm wary of looking up the drug on the internet), they say, "If you have to have a pain killer, this is probably the least dangerous." My functional medicine practitioner would like to get me off it eventually, but right now I prefer to stay with the devil I know. The only time I notice debilitating pain is, when at 6:00 p.m., I realize I've forgotten to take my last pill. The reminder may prove that I am addicted. If so, so be it. Gabapentin works quite well and provides me with an almost pain-free life. As Alex Trebek, host of *Jeopardy!* who had stage four pancreatic cancer, pointed out in his book, "Quality of life is important."

I could not be in this relatively comfortable relationship with chronic pain had I not complained and confronted my doctors with specific concerns. Above all, stay away from nice doctors who are ineffectual. Keep asking, probing, and asking again. Then . . . ask yet again.

I could not be in this relatively comfortable relationship with chronic pain had I not complained and confronted my doctors with specific concerns.

When you have a chronic and terminal disease, no one should tell you that you shouldn't take pain medication that works for you. It's *your* body, and taking ownership of treatment is an essential right. And that should apply, especially unto your final chapter.

I think of a cancer patient and friend of mine whose cervical cancer returned, and her physicians recommended another round of chemotherapy and surgery. She decided that she wanted to go into hospice and only take pain medication, such as morphine. When I asked about her decision, she said that her stage-four diagnosis put, "a membrane between me and the rest of the world." Patrice passed away in November 2018, leading her life as she wished into a peaceful death. I'm grieved at her loss—she was only fifty-seven—but I respect her wish not to suffer any more. Her perception of the foyer into her own death as a "membrane" between herself and others is an eloquent metaphor of what the terminal cancer patient can feel about living among the normal and healthy.

Very much among the living cancer patients, my friend, Allen, has tried other medications, but cannot keep the lifestyle he enjoys without oxycodone. The news reports of the opioid crisis is, indeed, frightening. Many people who don't have cancer but have other debilitating conditions have died because of these addictions. But, while I appreciate Allen's doctor trying CBD creams and other milder substances, I stand by Allen's decision to use whatever he needs to maintain his normal activity.

Allen, eighty-two, is a handsome, strapping guy with a great laugh, a lovely and smart girlfriend, a lively family, and a remarkable project to tell the story of his life in print. With no formal training in writing, in the last two years, this life-long engineer has written seven short books that tell fascinating stories about his religion, family, dramatic incidents, and his work and love lives. With each book in his series, The Sidewalk Philosopher, his prose style improves in clarity, grace, and wit. The books, printed by a local print house, stand proudly on his bookshelf amongst the many paintings on his walls. Oxycodone, he tells me, knocks him out for about an hour, and he must rest. But then he's good for the rest of the day. I celebrate his decision and his vitality through his choice of pain killers.

OTHER APPROACHES TO PAIN RELIEF

There are also some powerful mind-body approaches to alleviating pain. The most impressive, as mentioned earlier, is the Tibetan lama's story of the healing power of the mind. Through the discipline of meditation, the Buddhist lama Phakyab Rinpoche shared how he cured himself of gangrene in his right ankle. The great healing powers that lie within triumph in his dramatic story. Choosing compassion and courage, mind over matter, he teaches what is possible with intention, discipline, and spiritual strength.

Recently, I learned of the extraordinary power of Transcendental Meditation®. Buddhist monks take, on average, seven years to perfect pure consciousness. With training, TM practitioners can achieve this state within five minutes, according to a long time TM expert, Joseph H. Quaide, III. In deep sleep, which normally takes about five hours to achieve, oxygen absorption goes down about 8 percent. In Transcendental Meditation, oxygen is reduced about 16 percent. This state can be a powerhouse of healing for many ailments.

And Dr. Lissa Rankin, author of *Mind over Medicine*, reminds us of "the inner pilot light," and others speak of the power of meditation to lower stress, encourage the relaxation response and, therefore, mitigate or even eliminate pain. I have found meditation to be helpful with my back pain in the short term, but I needed something more powerful in order to be functional: to work at home, to walk in the City, to exercise, to travel, and to be an active citizen with others and my surroundings. Thus, I rely on pharmaceuticals with important ancillary help from acupuncture, meditation, and prayer.

I would encourage an exploration of other pain treatments, but you have to be disciplined enough to make the effort *while* you're suffering. The cannabis explosion is showing some promise of alleviating muscle pain, for example. And acupuncture has been known, after repeated treatments, to make a difference in back pain, arthritis distress, and other chronic conditions. Meditation, according to my acupuncture therapist, is the basis for all kinds of coping. "Go Within," said the Indian magician in teaching the young American magus the ultimate power of healing.

So much of pain maintains its mystery, but there are artful ways we can keep it at bay. I relish this story about those who would learn more about this bane of humanity:

A pain researcher and a vision expert were talking.

"You still don't know how pain works?" the vision guy asked the pain guy.

"You may know something about how vision works," the pain man replied, "how the retina's rods and cones receive light stimuli, how its nerve cells transmit them via the optic nerve to the brain, and so on. But tell me—in what part of the brain does beauty lie?"

The vision guy fell silent.

"Let me know when you find it," the pain man says, "because pain is right next door."

—— ✺ ——

Imelda Marcos's particular pain was insomnia, and her way of dealing with it reminds me of that other door. Imelda Marcos, along with her husband Ferdinand (who was ill for much of their reign, so Imelda really ran the country) ruled the Philippines for many years until a revolution finally brought the Marcoses to justice for misusing—to a spectacular extent—government funds. Ken was called in at the end of the process of liquidating their possessions. He was charged with selling their private plane and in particular, tracking down the art the Marcoses had purchased over the years. He discovered some interesting facts about the sumptuous lifestyle they had adopted and how they incorporated many others into their embezzlement of the Filipino treasury.

For example, Imelda lent Filipino money to her friends, who would then deposit it into banks and live off the interest. When she required the funds, they'd return part of the principle. Searching for these funds after the Marcos era ended was difficult.

This may have been because Imelda's mindset toward wealth was distinctive. When questioned by the authorities about her use of government funds for her lavish acquisitions, they asked how much money she really had.

"I don't know," she answered. "If you know how much money you have, you don't have very much, do you?"

Imelda had almost a mystical sense of treasure. It was an infinite or incalculable number creating a penumbra around her. She could just pluck at it and find enough in her hand to buy the next thing.

But there were other myths that grew around her that simply weren't true, like her shoes.

Imelda's famous shoe collection was not the result of her shopping, but the result of a tradition in the Philippines of certain guilds, a carry-over from the medieval times to assure excellence in craft. The shoemakers' guild had a ruling which required each craftsman who went from apprentice, to journeyman, to master, to make a great pair of shoes and give them to the chairperson of the guild. It so happened that Imelda was the chairperson, as she had been for many years. No wonder this was one crowded shoe closet!

But she was certainly extravagant in other ways. When the Pope visited, Imelda wanted to impress him, so she built an entire ideal village in the Philippines with his personal cell made of pineapple and decorated with exquisite pineapple cloth, pinya or piña, the queen of fabric in the Philippines.

And the Marcoses had many homes. One was in New York, a townhouse decorated with huge pictures of famous people. After the Marcoses' fall from government, the new Filipino administration sold the townhouse to recoup some of the millions squandered by the previous rulers, including the art. But the new government wouldn't allow the pictures of the American Presidents that grace the walls to be sold. In the portrait of Ronald Reagan, he appeared eight feet tall, wearing many fictitious medals across his chest on a big ribbon. President Carter, on the contrary, was only a half-figure. The Filipino government was embarrassed and wouldn't allow these portraits—or Imelda's shoes—to be auctioned.

Near the end of the auction, Ken managed to buy some of Imelda's linens. The bed linens and tablecloths were made of piña, the glorious pineapple thread that felt like silk. It was the fabric of the aristocrats, and I enjoyed its luxury. The sheets were soft and lush, but the tablecloths were even more precious. Called *piña calado*, they were encrusted with the most spectacular embroidery. We slept under the sheets for years until they fell apart with laundering. I made a lovely dress out of one of the tablecloths. But after a few years, it became very fragile.

I have one tablecloth left. I dream of using it for a granddaughter's sixteenth birthday. Will I have a granddaughter? Will I be alive?

The most intriguing story Ken shared about Imelda Marcos was the way she handled her pain of insomnia. She'd call the Director of the National Ballet at 3:00 a.m. to come to her home and dance for her. In the islands, she hired "Blue Ladies" who would read to her all night. But in New York, she installed a karaoke nightclub on the top floor of her townhouse where she invited friends and encouraged the parties that lasted until 4:00 a.m. Her favorite song was "The Yellow Rose of Texas," and she sang it all the time. One of the famous escorts who was frequently seen at Imelda's nightclub was the actor George Hamilton, who must have demonstrated nocturnal resilience. Other party goers tried to leave before her 4:00 a.m. farewell. One account had them crawling across the floor to get to the exit; Imelda was engrossed in her own performance.

Imelda faced her pain—insomnia—with extravagant artfulness. It would seem that for her, the pain door was indeed, right next to beauty. For Imelda, an accessible and always affordable escape.

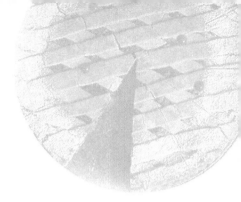

10 THOUGHTS OF DEATH

The most beautiful experience we can have is the mysterious.
It is the source of all true art and all true science.
Whoever does not know it, who can no longer pause to stop
in wonder or stand rapt in awe, is as good as dead.

—Albert Einstein

Maybe I should have called this chapter "Wrestling with the Angel."

The effort it takes to embrace the imminence of death and the need to face the fear, pain, loneliness, and grief of disease—yet still find the glory and joy of living every day—and to keep loving our darlings—*this* is the contest.

Acute simultaneity is wrestling with the Angel. It can be a strenuous, fascinating struggle. Never boring, never without rewards, and for me, it always leads to wisdom.

At some point, give death serious thought. It is part of living.

Ram Dass reminds us about maintaining spiritual development and why turning inward is good for us. "The ego, this incarnation, is life and dying. The soul is infinite." Anne Lamott, in *Almost Everything: Notes on Hope*, wrote a remarkable essay about death that I envy. She talks about our probable first discovery of death with our pets: "they stop wriggling." And then into our twenties and thirties we are terrified, but we must truly look at the grimace of the dead face, stay bedside with the dying, even prepare their bodies for the grave.

"The reason to draw close to death when we're younger is to practice finding and living in the soul. This grows our muscles for living. . . . We see that the soul was right here all along, everywhere, and consequently we can once again feel charmed by the world," says Lamott.

Death and being charmed by the world equal acute simultaneity.

—∞—

There is so much Asian art in our home that, when I first moved in, I thought I was in a men's club, or a never-ending scene from the opera, *Madame Butterfly*. So, in my courtship with Ken, I finagled a trip to Mexico for us, strategically planning a counterbalance to all those Chinese and Japanese woodcuts, paintings, sculpture; all the Guanyins, Tibetan prayer objects, jade, and porcelain. Yikes!

The trip to San Miguel d'Allende bathed us in a radically different culture for ten days.

And it worked! We came home with a new mission. During my chemotherapy, we remodeled the upstairs into a Mexican suite: all the vibrant colors—reds and greens and teals—the buoyant patterns of the tiles, the parrots, and woven art. We even have an amazingly colored ceramic toilet. My stepdaughter calls it, "A party for your butt." And when you walk into the adjacent bedroom, you can almost hear the mariachi band!

But downstairs . . . ah, there are those reminders of a quieter, stranger world.

I would like you to examine the most striking object— the *kapala*, the skull of a monk treated like a work of art, a "vessel of inestimable value" in our living room. The Tibetan monks select a particular monk who has proven to be holy in his lifetime and has followed the regimen of Buddhism, so as to be a model of goodness, compassion, and peace. When he passes and the body has decayed and the flesh has dissolved, they remove the skull. The first stage is complete.

This next ritual proves that the living monks have chosen the right skull: a monk pisses into the hollow head until the right tone is heard. When the sound is right, when it's determined that *this* skull is to become the sacred vessel, the second stage is complete, and the transformation of the skull into the holy *kapala* begins.

First, the bone is burnished until it shines. Then silver is molded and carved into the teeth and attached to the upper and lower jaw. Small coins are shaped into the eye sockets. An ornate top is created so that when the *kapala* is upside down, this cap can be removed to reveal the cavity within awaiting the ceremonial substances. The total effect is startling and beautiful, as if the head has become a royal presence. Sometimes, as with our *kapala*, a stand is created so that the skull sits in it, signaling more its function as a vessel than as the icon of death.

Kapala points to the illegality of collecting human skulls and the enduring attraction of what, to some, has been considered works of art.

Related to this art object in our living room is Colin Dickey's fascinating book, *Cranioklepty*, which describes a deep-seated enchantment with the pursuit of genius through a new science during the Age of Enlightenment: phrenology. The major proponent of phrenology, Dr. Franz Joseph Gall, believed that great artistic or scientific achievement would be evident on the outside of the skull. Like the gravediggers of Egypt, Gall and his followers believed that the mystery of the human condition could be unveiled through the head alone.

Dickey traces the "skullduggery" of the nineteenth century when certain collectors stole the skulls of famous artists and statesmen. The heads of Haydn, Mozart, Beethoven, and Napoleon were involved in this ghoulish pursuit because their skulls could command huge sums of money. Lincoln's skull was pursued over countless attempts so that that his corpse was finally exhumed and buried in concrete. Of course, phrenology has been debunked, and the secrets of genius were never exposed by the objective evidence of the bones.

As Dickey puts it triumphantly, "The definition of genius could never be articulated by the skull, but by the art created: the music, the writing of the brain within." The *kapala* reminds us that it is the mind—wider than the sky—as Emily Dickinson says, and not the skull that holds it, outlining our world, our capacious lives.

What we leave behind is an extension of that mind, which is well beyond the confines of our bones. Whether it is art, or money, or a library, we should see the legacy as a triumph over death.

Now, what will be *your* legacy?

AWE AND WONDER

Another solution—another venture away from thoughts of death—is the pursuit of wonder, especially with a certain kind of magic, a craft, and mystery with which I've become enraptured in the last few years. Perhaps I am drawn to *wonder* as the ultimate antidote to this life's ending. It's a kind of precursor—an exercise in attention, a practice leap—to the spiritual life. No wonder David Abram calls it "a natural, wild, irrepressible force within human nature."

In his book, *Here Is Real Magic: A Magician's Search for Wonder in the Modern World*, Nate Staniforth sees that magic is indifferently accepted today, whereas earlier, it was an essential part of life, an ambassador between the tribe and the environment. The magician worked on the balance between the community and the rain, the earth, the forest, the world. The magician was like the negotiator for the fishermen as they did dangerous tasks, like fishing in the ocean, not in the safe lagoon. Real magic was part of a happy life. Nowadays, they are illusionists, not magicians, Las Vegas bound.

Perhaps, magic is a kind of referee in the struggle between the thoughts of life and death. Magic, awe, and wonder tells us that we cannot know everything, and we certainly cannot know the full meaning of either life or death.

I think of the Indian magus in Nate Staniforth's description of "the street magicians of Shadipur Depot" below:

In a small village in one of India's poorest neighborhoods, the Shadipur Depot, a crowd has gathered around a boy and his father. The son is blindfolded while his father sharpens a sword with a stone.

While the villagers watch as if in a trance, the man raises his sword and massacres the boy. The butchery is quick and expert, and the man is calm.

The boy's body, broken, and bleeding is in the center of the crossroads. His blood runs to meet the feet of those who watch, and they must step aside to avoid the streams.

The father takes a cloth and gathers up the ruined body in the cloth. He is tender, and he folds the edges carefully over the small bundle. The villagers see the blood seeping through the weave of the cloth.

He paces around the body in a circle and whispers harsh and determined words. Then he shouts in a strange language as his hand is outstretched toward his son.

The cloth over the boy's body begins to move. It falls away and the boy emerges, totally unharmed, or surely back from the dead!

His wounds are not there. He is perfectly whole and healthy. The father raises his hands in triumph.

The boy smiles and takes a bow.

Stunning, heartbreaking, heart healing. I believe that we will never be the same after seeing this magic, even if only in our mind's eye.

In modern life, most people find magic an experience for kids' birthday parties, or—like this story from the Shadipur Depot—a scary devil-worship, cult-like trick. But, as Ingrid Fetell Lee, persuades in *The Aesthetics of Joy*, magic is essential. "At the root of our love of rainbows, comets, and fireflies is the belief that our world is bigger and more amazing than we ever dreamed it could be." For those of us who feel our hold on life is fragile, we might very well pursue this source of joy and mystery.

For example, the scientific experiment at UCLA. The seniors were tested before and after viewing the Grand Canyon, which proved that our biochemistry changes when we witness a spectacular monument. The good cytokines increase—those soldiers in our blood stream that fight infection. Wonder bolsters our immune system.

Wonder can not only improve our health; it is also the vector to enchantment.

Matthew Hutson, author of *The 7 Laws of Magical Thinking: How Irrational Beliefs Keep Us Happy, Healthy, and Sane,* tells us that magic comforts us with a more profound sense of meaning, "Magic fights the cold sense that we're alone in the universe."

It shows us that the "universe is looking out for us." He cites research that confirms magical thinking generates not only optimism about the future, but also recovery from devastating events. Those who believe in magic find more pleasure in life than those who are skeptical. Magic gives meaning and, therefore, ignites our sense of spirituality, whether religious or not.

SPIRIT

September 29, 2019, 10:00 a.m., watching *CBS Sunday Morning:*

I rarely watch this show, but this day something nudged me to make my kale chips for breakfast and eat while sitting before the TV while Ken was settling down to work.

Olivia Newton-John was talking about her stage-four breast cancer, which had returned in her bones. The interviewer, Gayle Smith, asked her about the prognosis.

"I don't talk about that. I know the life expectancy that medicine often gives, but I don't believe that will apply to me. So, I don't talk about it." She smiled.

Gayle asked her, "Do you think about death?"

"I try not to," she said, "but of course I think about it. All of us must face it somehow. I could be hit by a tree and die. But I believe am going to live a long time."

I was stunned by her parallel philosophy to my own, and I also felt that Mom's spirit had nudged me to sit down and watch this segment of a TV show that I don't usually see.

Whether or not you believe in spirits, ghosts, the afterlife, or angels, you can attribute something to your mysterious unconscious, intuition, or the life force within you. This won't work for everyone. But if you can believe that this present reality is not the only one; that some force or agent is beyond what you can see, then comfort awaits. It has for me.

Full disclosure for why I have faith in the beyond: my Catholic upbringing—kindergarten through college—

grounded me in the deep culture of the church: the liturgy, the saints, hymns and especially Holy Communion. Although I am what is called "a fallen away Catholic," I still can't forget that I wanted to be a nun when I was seven or eight. (My mother put the kibosh on that idea). I've always been drawn to the mystery of the silent, locked away Carmelites who have little or no contact with the world. (My friends break into hilarity when they think about me as a recluse banished from consignment shops and parties forever!)

But the spiritual education runs deep. In the pocket of my Volkswagen is a plastic relief of Mother Mary—a prize for my penmanship in the eighth grade! I've kept it as a talisman in my car since I started to drive. On its back is the date, 1956.

When I was first diagnosed with breast cancer, I went to see a holy man in the Bronx who guided me through prayer in a special chapel. During the blessings, I felt what seemed to be a kiss on my right cheek. Brother Bart was yards away at the altar. I was overwhelmed with the sense of love coming from above, and I trembled and wept, tipping my head backward toward what I thought was the source of such sweetness. It only lasted for a few moments, but it is forever in my memory. Even Brother Bart was surprised, and he asked me, with amazement, many questions about the experience.

When I was first diagnosed with breast cancer, I went to see a holy man in the Bronx who guided me through prayer in a special chapel.

Anyway—a mystical experience. I treasure the thought as a piece of precious jewelry, more magnificently dear than the Mother Mary plaque in the pocket of my Volkswagen.

One way to de-fang thoughts of death and answer the yearning for the lost one is to believe in ghosts. I'm a shameless proponent of this belief. Whenever a friend loses a loved one, I send them a note and ask them to "look for their lost one in their lives. They may become a daily beauty." Look for their presence in small things, I urge. Daddy is, I swear, with me in the car, especially in driving emergencies. And my mother's spirit responds when I misplace items.

"Mom, where did I put that pair of pink earrings I wore the other day?" Sure enough, they turn up in the bathroom. Silly? Perhaps, but a comfort, nonetheless.

As Anne Lamott says, our dead ones "visit—ectoplasmically—and you invite them to come closer."

Don't hesitate to move toward whatever religion you're drawn to. Chapels, synagogues, priests, rabbis, teachers of Buddhism. Spiritual comfort comes in many forms.

Recently, at a ladies' luncheon, when it was my turn, a psychic told me I was a "faerie." Not an angel, mind you, a faerie. Angels are different. They have big muscles. In storms, they watch over huge airplanes with grandmothers traveling from New York to grandsons in California. I always think of those angels like the geese in the movie my brother made years ago, *Fly Away Home*. The cinematographer somehow came right up close to those birds and let us see the strenuous effort of their work in flight. Geese breathe hard as they move those wings. So do angels, I imagine, those powerful athletes of the air, protecting the flying steel I sit in while I silently pray for the Los Angeles airport, our safe landing, and Mac Weaver rummaging in my carry-on for his first present.

Faeries, also called "elementals," have slender bodies. They wear a lot of filmy material. Gossamer and smoke encircle their tiny physiques. Little breezes tell you they are there. Their hands are especially lovely, with long fingers. I had those as an infant . . . a telltale sign of my faerie-dom.

Angels hover around soldiers in war and help you through childbirth. They wake up drivers falling asleep on lonely country roads. They keep your purse away from the thief who would steal it when you go to the ladies' room.

Faeries move the paint brush, so the stroke of watercolor is perfect. Most of all, they help make you pretty. In the eighteenth-century poem, "The Rape of the Lock," Alexander Pope creates Arabella Fermor, who has lots of faeries at her toilette. Dusting her perfect cheeks, putting a stray curl into its proper place, banishing too much rouge. A little cluster of them sit on her exquisite ears to keep her hairdo tidy.

Faeries like to hang out at Sephora and cosmetic counters in department stores. In the climb to be a true angel, I think of them as what I once was—a doctoral candidate for a PhD. Quite a gauntlet! First you must pass many graduate classes, then take terrifying tests called comprehensives, and THEN write a long book which is ratified by scary professors who may not even like the damn thing. Faeries, I surmise, didn't quite get past the comprehensive tests. (These candidates are called with scorn by some "ABD's"—"all but the dissertation.") They are pre-angels, not failed ones, not demoted certainly. They are wanna-be angels, but in the meantime, they are possibly writing their scholarly book in their spare time and being charming helpers and helpers of charm.

Some say, they are also "keepers of health concerns." I'll cling to that serious one of their duties and smile at my make-up brush as I apply just the right amount of coral to my cheek.

So much we don't know! In *Mind Over Medicine,* Lissa Rankin claims a different magic in the placebo effect. Again and again, she shows how patients who *believe* they will live and thrive do just that. And those who are told that they have only a few weeks or months to live, die within those weeks and months. As the poet, Marianne Moore, has written,

> "The mind is an enchanted thing
> Like the glaze on a katydid's wing
> Subdivided by sun
> Till the nettings are legion."
> *and*
> "Wonders will never cease, as long as we are willing to look for them."—Eden Phillpotts

—◈—

This story is the opposite of a respectful salute to the deceased, who clearly had no faeries about. I include it for its humor.

The police raided a mafia crook's house. Because of IRS debt, the cops confiscated all his art. Fat Arnie, an associate of the mafia guy, complained and said that some of the stuff belonged to him. Ken was brought in to sort Arnie's collection from that of the mafia man. In the process, Ken got rather friendly with the talkative Arnie, who told him this tale of how he liked to enjoy himself.

First, he would get his "boot" (booth) at conferences (usually gun shows). Then he would buy a bottle of "hootch," procure a prostitute and then a local hotel room. One time, he confided to Ken, he and his female companion got hungry after a few drinks, so they ordered Chinese. After the meal arrived and they enjoyed it, they both fell asleep in the bed. Arnie awoke later to find red goo all over the sheets. He panicked at what he thought was a bloody mess: "I thought I ate her!!" Instead, of course, it was the Moo Goo Gai Pan mashed into the sleeping duo's bedsheets.

Later, Fat Arnie died after a liposuction procedure went bad. Ken also worked on that estate appraisal because Arnie's wife remembered him from the earlier IRS project. When Ken expressed his condolences and regret that he could not attend the funeral, he said, "I hope it was well-attended and that it was arranged as he wished."

His wife answered, "Arnie was so full of shit that I could have given him an enema and buried him in a shoebox."

Death is around the corner. Even as Arnie planned a thinner, more attractive self, fate dealt him a cruel hand.

And yet, death is not the only fear. I've found that surprising horrors lurk around me, reminding me that the monster is still there when I haven't thought about it in some time. Like soldiers who hide in trees to kill the unsuspecting enemy, they ambush you with hit-and-run tactics. Here's how to blunt their impact.

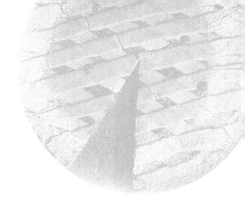

GUERILLA ATTACKS

Death is the sound of distant thunder at a picnic.

—W. H. Auden

There are the sudden incidents that ambush you: stories you're told, advertisements on TV, casual or intentional comments, unexpected horrors that pop up and bite you.

Your shoemaker tells you his mother just died of metastatic cancer. She was fifteen years younger than you.

You stumble across a website that shows the life expectancy of people with stage-four cancer. It isn't long.

An ad comes on the TV about the "new normal" when taking IBRANCE®, which made you deathly ill. When you hear the list of side effects, you have to leave the room.

You go to a meeting in the City and someone tells you the story about another cancer patient diagnosed with metastatic cancer. "A great guy. Lived a full life and we loved him," she says cheerfully. Later, I go back to her and can't resist asking, "How did he die?" "Oh, the cancer finally caught up with him."

When I pay for a short consultation, a famous holistic doctor tells me that he knew someone who had metastatic cancer, and "she lived four years." I'm in year three.

There's a book by Nancy Riggs, who wrote of metastatic breast cancer. When diagnosed, her husband said to her, "Can't wait to get back to normal . . ." You find out that she died before her book was published.

I got a phone call from Kara in Baltimore who told me about her triple-negative breast cancer. When she asked the doctor too many questions, he screamed at her, "You will be dead in a year."

Dark voices. Here's how my thoughts race after a guerilla attack like the ones above:

My back hurt that morning. Not so bad, but it hurt, and I wondered about the results of my most recent PET scan. I'd had it the day before, and I knew that they'd shot me with radioactive liquid and watched where the fluid went. It follows the sugar. That's the place where the cancer is. I stare at the box of Dunkin Donuts Ken has brought in. The radioactivity was still in me. It had only been thirty hours.

They told me I couldn't be with children under two years old. If I were in LA, I couldn't be with Mac Weaver who loves to share delight with me. Delight: my chief quality. It makes up for a lot. Mac and I share this trait in deep measure. When two-year-old Mac first met the little machine that, when you turn the knob, a plastic bubble comes out with a tiny toy inside, he looked at the surprise in his hand, and I could see a slight electric shock go through him. That's delight, that's wonder—a visceral kick that reminds us that we don't know it all, and what we don't know is liable to be wonderful. When his mother plays a trick on him and puts the fork full of food in *her* mouth, not his, he laughs and turns to look at me to share the fun. That is life.

That's delight, that's wonder—a visceral kick that reminds us that we don't know it all, and what we don't know is liable to be wonderful.

But the mild pain in my back is death. That's a guerilla attack.

That morning I looked at my Rockettes—the hanging baskets of petunias and begonias on my garden wall. The way they are angled away from me makes me think of the famous chorus line at Radio City Music Hall: precise and gorgeous, legs as flowers. They bloom outside the kitchen window, each with their portion of sun and shade. I wept with thankfulness that I was still alive yet feared that my time may be short.

But then I turned from the sink and wandered into my living room, where the dancing gods in brass statues are backlit by big windows overlooking acres of wetlands. Ken's office is next to this remarkable arrangement. When I showed up at his door, he invited me in to look at another beautiful thing—this time on his computer screen. A client wanted an appraisal for a gift to a famous museum: it was a Russian cassock—or gown—worn only by the highest

Russian Orthodox bishops, an encrusted liturgical robe with pearls, rubies, emeralds, and fantastic embroidery. I am fascinated immediately by the close-ups of the workmanship of this priceless work of art. There are tiny faces emerging on the cloth and they are barely an inch big. Each face has an expression made by silver or gold thread.

The guerilla impact fades from my heart when Ken tells me the story of how this *Assael Sakkos* was made: patient nuns spent years learning the craftsmanship, probably in the Kremlin workshops of the seventeenth century. Because I used to sew my own clothes when I was a teenager, I had a flash of sympathy for those young and old women bending over the gorgeous Italian fabric. Some apparently only sewed the faces. Other worked the jewels into the cloth. There were pomegranates set in rubies. Foliage was created out of dense clusters of gold, emerald, and diamonds. Forty-one thousand pearls were in one cassock from the period.

So heavy was this encrusted style that when a chalice cover was made—only about a foot square-—and the officiant took the cover from the assistant and turned to put it on the altar, a breeze was created when the heavy fabric of the cassock moved. So, it was called the *Vozdukh*, "the breeze" in Russian. Those who sat in the front row of the cathedral waited in suspense for that blessing from the sweeping gesture of a priest holding a crafted chalice cover that was simply out of this world.

But wearing the big garment!!! Pity the bishops! Those who walked down the long cathedral aisle carried many pounds of bejeweled robe and fought the exhaustion of long Orthodox services. Could this be a recompense for the pain of the sedulous nuns who were sometimes literally blinded by their devotion to liturgical grandeur?

Nothing in this art is done in a panic; no one succumbs to guerilla attacks to create such beauty. When my heart stops suddenly in one of these episodes, I must remember the *Assael Sakkos* and the glacially slow attention of those nuns who created a magnificent tapestry.

VISIT OLD PHOTOGRAPHS

Are scrap books trending? No wonder! I discovered this exploration into the past when a friend asked me to find a picture of her husband, who I'd known for many years. I had to paw through old albums in a terrible disorganized mess, and, in the process, found myself enchanted with pictures of me when I was sixteen, thirty-five, fifty, sixty-two, sixty-five.

And pictures of my husband, skinnier, my escort at galas, parties in the City, on the Queen Mary II, Queen Elizabeth, Viking Sun, in Lisbon, and the Caribbean islands. Do you know what I discovered?

I HAVE HAD A WONDERFUL, FULL, AND GLORIOUS LIFE!!!!!!!!!!

This thought also calms me from the guerilla attacks.

I have a few old-fashioned albums and a couple of wicker boxes full of pictures not kept in any particular time frame or topic, although some of the albums are individually devoted to special vacations.

When I'm feeling a little blue, worried, or just plain sad, I like to go into the wicker boxes because it offers surprises—sometimes from long ago. No order means a higgeldy-piggeldy cornucopia of my history. Pictures of my boys, now handsome men at forty and thirty-seven, here they are at three years old, at ten, as infants. These would be next to a scene of a party I threw for myself turning fifty: I am alone and wearing a sequined dress, sitting thoughtfully, holding a scotch and ignoring my guests for a few minutes while somebody snapped this aging, but still attractive, single parent and thinker. And here's one of my mother holding my son David at fifteen months—she is smiling slightly, the face of the besotted grandmother taking time out of her Florida retirement to savor grandsons. Oh, and here's one of Ken and I when he was wooing me about a dozen years ago—one of the many selfies he would take of us around the world—this one in a Mexican restaurant, our heads leaning hard against each other in front of a wildly colorful background, our grins the flower of new love. My eldest son's wedding with my brother as officiant; laughter and deep affection entwined throughout the ritual; a delicious one of my two-year-old grandson, walking with gusto in his scuffed tiny sneakers, a Lambie doll dangling from a fat little fist, smiling into his future, enchanting me, and making me understand my own mother's smile in the earlier photograph. And there's Ken and I in front of the massive ship on the dock in Turkey; with friends on the top deck of the *Cunard* with the Romanian bartender; of me doing the three little pigs in an improv class with RADA actors on board; me in a fox coat saluting the retreating dock in Brooklyn with a champagne toast!

When I'm feeling a little blue, worried or just plain sad, I like to go into the wicker boxes . . .

Wonderful reminders of a rich, full life. *How dare you be sad, downhearted, or pitiful with all these joyful, precious moments—inhaled, absorbed. And no one can take them away!*

Do it! Get out your old albums and feel sorry for everyone who has their precious photos on their phones.

REAL PAINTINGS ARE DELICATE

A company in Columbia, Indiana, hired Ken to determine the cause of damage to an Ellsworth Kelly painting worth millions. The large painting hung six inches from a secretary's desk. The painting was lemon gold throughout, but there was a brownish black swath across the bottom that shouldn't have been there. How did this happen?

Ken watched the secretary and the painting. A Chinese girl with very long hair answered the phone, and each time she reached for the phone, she swung her long hair across the painting. Thus, the brunette discoloration. Although Ken is a master conservator, he could not fix the painting which was forever marred by the oils and unguents in the beautiful, sweeping hair of the woman answering the phone.

As for surprise reminders of death, like panic attacks . . . you can fight back! You can't eliminate guerilla attacks, but you can dissolve them like lumps in a cake batter, or if you are aggressive, kill them with a fly swatter.

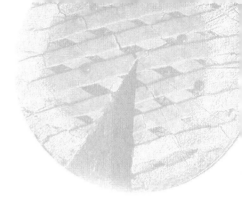

GETTING STUCK IN A CANCER PATIENT IDENTITY

It takes courage to grow up and become who you really are.

—e. e. cummings

Fascinating for me—Ken's small footprint compared to my large one. He never leaves much trash, just a bit of paper in the bathroom waste can.

Even his napkins after dinner are always clean. After any meal, he can fold a pristine cloth. His car interior is impeccable. His clothes never smell, even after heavy labor. Things taken to the cleaners don't need service. His skin is white and without smell. My first husband had a distinct aroma that was sometimes strong. Ken is like a prince or a saint in his skin. He cooks with a surgeon's tidiness, clearing up after himself as he works so that at any point in the process, the kitchen looks almost unused.

Is this a gender thing? Women are so used to messes, we thrive on moist endpapers of projects, meals, creation. Ancient texts tell us that the world was in the beginning, after all, chaos, largely water and earth, leavened with air, heated with fire. Look at the drain in the kitchen sink. It could be the stuff of a new earth, or the fertilized egg, not quite yet a zygote.

The true occupation for a woman is the watery indistinguishable mess of everyday: the stew that must be prepared, shaped, cleaned, smoothed, spiced, cooked, above all—handled.

I am the Dionysian mess to Ken's Apollonian order: the steamfitter's daughter to the Scandinavian prince; the color to the line; the flesh to the bone; the dancer to the dance.

—⟋∿⟍—

Embedded in the perspective of a terminal disease is the opportunity to discover our authenticity. If not now, when will we find and define our true selves? The glorious individuality of our tastes, preferences, habits, styles—warts and all!

Age really pushes us toward this authenticity, but I wish I had found it earlier. I find that I dress with more flash and glamour than I did twenty years ago. Having become an expert buyer in thrift shops, I enjoy the diversity of the merchandise and, with the divining rod of my own personal style, I choose items others might ignore. Fashion can be fun, especially when you're on a tight budget and the choices before you are all eligible for that skinny column of figures.

"What the hell," I might say, "I could use this short dress with black fringe for a Halloween party! Plus, it's only eight bucks and it fits!"

Perhaps the best example of my authentic code shows up at my cosmetics table. I wear makeup every morning of my life. I was taught this early when I recovered from a great grief—my first husband leaving me for a younger woman when I had just given birth.

At that terrible time, my friend, Marjorie, listened to me weep yet another time on the phone and stopped me.

"Carole, go to the bathroom and put on foundation, eye makeup, and lipstick."

Numb, I obeyed. And like magic, my black mood turned to gray and then polka dot and then pink.

From that day to this—four decades later—I follow this same regimen that gives me the face I choose—*my* face, not the face of an abandoned wife, an exhausted single parent, a worried mother, a breast cancer patient—or now, the face of metastatic cancer. As the sign proclaimed while we were driving through Hamburg, Ontario, Canada: "We cannot cure the world of sorrow, but we can choose to live in joy."

Getting rid of certain mental habits is key to finding your authentic self. Shame is a big one. Banishing shame—a common reflex when you judge your thoughts and actions—will uncover your essence, psychologists say. Another, less intense, but more pervasive demon is self-doubt. Second guessing your tastes, your impulses, your predilections, oh

I've been there! Self-doubt stymies creativity, serenity and, certainly, confidence.

Getting rid of certain mental habits is key to finding your authentic self.

—ഗഗ—

Laura Carfang, creator of the website survivingbreastcancer. org, has a wonderful riff on self-doubt, and I share it with you with her permission:

I want to flip self-doubt on its head. Actually, to be blunt, I want to smash it against the wall! I don't know why I am plagued with this ingrained mentality. We could go on to psychoanalyze my childhood and the numerous events that happened during 3rd grade. . . . Or we could log onto Zoom, sip our delectable coffee (Nespresso), and contemplate which wave of feminism we belong to and the various social constructs that have perpetuated self-doubt since the beginning of time.

Cut off my breast, lose my hair, inject my body with the most toxic chemicals imaginable—all to "Save the Tatas?" Of course, my self-confidence is going to take a blow! I may look fine and dandy on the outside, but I pretty much have a breakdown anytime I have to buy a new dress or find a swimsuit for the summer. I ended up donating all my beautiful silk blouses that I used to wear to work because we all know silk and hot flashes do not go hand and hand. While colleagues take time off to go to the dentist, I am taking time off to get infusions. It's a constant reminder of cancer, but I refuse to let this diagnosis cast aspersions."

Constant reminders of cancer must be banished by faith in the future and confidence that life will still hold other beauties than silk blouses.

—◦◦◦◦—

When I think of confidence, blind confidence, I think of the delicious short scenes of King George III of England in the musical *Hamilton.* While the rebels are building a nation, he appears from the wings of the stage in full royal regalia—crown and red velvet cape with ermine—and he conveys his scorn for the Americans.

His melodic song touches on the tea party and not-so-veiled threats of his anger. He reminds the rebels that they "belong" to him, and that "oceans rise; empires fall." That is, in the cycles of nature and history, this relationship between the colonies and England is permanent. He rips away the veils off the threats, with images of armed battalions and the death of friends and family which will come in war.

Regal and warlike, the character is still comically wonderful. I also think he makes us hanker for such a strong, if obtuse, identity. King George's self-congratulation is enviable.

Of course, his regal tone has nothing to do with right or wrong. We know the king is a tyrant from the point of view of the Americans. It's his confidence that's still somehow winning and instructive: *"I will kill your friends and family to remind you of my love."*

Behold another path to authenticity. When we witness strong self-regard, self-definition, we might ask ourselves *What do I like?* and *"What am I like?* (in contrast to this person).

Gary Zukav defines "authentic power" as that which happens when your personality serves—becomes fully aligned with—the energy of your soul.

Met someone like that?

Here's a story I love for the very personal contrasting ways of regarding books—all of which are legitimate and passionate. Which of these types are you?

Consider the most famous and exclusive club for book collectors in New York City: members do not read the books but celebrate the binding and the typography. One member buys a watch owned by an iconic nineteenth writer of short stories. She pays $250,000 for a timekeeper that does not run. However, she would never fix it because the new pieces required to make it work would cause it to lose its authenticity.

Ken gave a book to a client who hurt her hand. He came back to find she had torn the book in two, so she could easily hold it in her good hand for reading. He was shocked.

Ken is a bibliophile with 20,000 books in his libraries. He also does not necessarily read them. But he gets great pleasure from *owning* them. I am a doctorate in English who is embarrassed if I don't read the books I acquire. My bookshelf shows battered favorites.

Then there is my friend, Nancy: she reads books and then gives them away!

All are book lovers.

Part of knowing ourselves is to discover what truly moves us—whether it is the art of surrendering to what you find intensely beautiful; or listening to your body as it responds to music; perhaps eloquent language; or what resonates for you in a museum. Will you read the book, tear it in two, or give it away? Ask, "What is my truth?"

Oceans rise; empires fall. Whether we are right or wrong, on the side of good taste or not, a Tory or a rebel, a thriver from disease or one closer to death, we can all be kings of our own souls.

ANOTHER HEALING HABIT

Seek out experiences of beauty, especially the sublime, a clear flight path to self-definition.

Adam Gopnik, in his book *Winter,* analyzes the appeal of the sublime as a strong response to that which is not simply beautiful, but offers the full span of human sympathy. "Oceans and thunderstorms, precipices, and abysses, towering volcanoes and above all snow-capped mountains . . . they outdo beauty because they frighten us, fill us with fear, with awe . . . and the mystery of the world."

The *sublime* is the big bruising brother of *wonder*. I still remember the first time I saw the Alps in my early twenties. Sitting in the passenger seat with my boyfriend in a sports car on a rainy day in southern Germany, I had no warning of what was ahead. Suddenly there it was, my first real mountain. I burst into tears with the magnificence and surprise. Strange, but I felt *hurt* somehow, as if "How could this be? Who kept this from me?"

My last trip on a cruise this past year was also full of heart-stopping moments seeing the Chilean Fjords, especially glaciers up close, volcanoes, waterfalls, and the great forests of Patagonia. But nothing can match that first Alpine vision. It left me with a yearning for the majestic power of nature. The sublime expands the soul, and for a flashing moment, shows us a towering mystery, and—with an aching stretch— the widest span of our heart.

Destruction of art in this story has a *sublime horrific* aspect.

Art collector, Trammel Crowe, was a millionaire real estate developer and passionate collector of east Asian art. Ken was asked to appraise his spectacular collection of Chinese jade carvings.

Afterward, his attractive wife, Margaret, came under the spell of a local preacher who convinced her that the jades were evil signs of the devil. (My husband's first wife had the same reaction to our Tibetan and Chinese statues in the living room. For her, the daughter of a Methodist preacher, she could not tolerate their images, reminding her of pagan rituals.) I can only surmise Mrs. Crowe's reaction to an apparently charismatic preacher. During a ritual offering, perhaps exorcising evil, the preacher took the jades out in a boat with the wife on the Crowes' man-made lake. While he read from the Bible, he smashed the jades and threw the pieces into the water.

So, Trammel hired Ken to rebuild his collection. After his death years later, his wife seemed to experience a productive contrition. She became the caretaker and curator of Trammel's renewed massive art collection, installing many of the pieces in a famous hotel in Dallas called the Anatole. She continued to visit the galleries every week to see that the collection was well cared for. Mrs. Crowe passed away in 2014.

Destroying the art and then rebuilding a spectacular collection? Mrs. Crowe, for reasons we will never know, changed her mind about art, even pagan art. The result is a breathtaking assembly of beauty from all over the world.

Mrs. Crowe, we can say, transformed her identity from a smasher of pagan art to a sophisticated collector of priceless objects.

In *The Moment of Lift*, Melinda Gates traces the process of changing a company from an aggressive, yelling, fighting, madly competitive male group at Microsoft to a passionate, courageous, and effective group of women who performed the work they loved.

Gates changed the culture of the workplace and the efficiency and vitality that was based on traditional masculine tendencies. She encouraged the women in this tech company to be creative and focused in a different way. I suggest we change the culture of fighting this disease similarly. Discover and be your authentic self, and that will be a leap in the right direction. Refuse to be the face of illness!

FORGERY

Of all Ken's adventures in art crime, perhaps the most colorful are the forgery stories—cautionary tales about how precious authenticity is and how fragile. Determining authenticity is perhaps the foundational skill of the appraiser. After all, the difference between the real thing and the fake can be the difference between two bucks and two million. Taxes, estate or otherwise, auction prices, divorce settlements, sales prices, or insurance awards all hinge on the gavel of the appraiser's estimated value.

But the appraiser can be hoodwinked. And these are the smartest criminals.

Whether it is the tale of the composite painting of the Russian artist, Fernand Leger, which ended in the murder of the owner, or the one about the two defrocked priests who created a fortune in tax deductions with manufactured masterpieces, the talent and brilliance of the crooks fascinate us. When we hear the tale of foolery, we say, "Who *are* these guys?"

The most striking and memorable forgery, for me, is the Ghost Army of World War II. Hundreds of artists used visual, sonic, and radio with audacious creativity to fool the Germans into believing battalions were waiting to fight. For example, inflatable tanks, sound effects, and rubber dummies impersonated whole divisions for making the enemy believe that D-Day would occur not at Normandy, but at the Pas de Calais. As written in *The Ghost Army of World War II* by Rick Sayles and Elizabeth Beyer, the Germans fell for it, and thus, thousands of lives were saved. These men of the 23rd Headquarters Special Troops and other divisions were artists who pretended—through stagecraft and a kind of magic— to be the US Army, and thereby, for example, protected Patton's infantry, which waited behind their subterfuge. These "forgers for the light" took their own lives into their hands in order to perform a remarkable service.

Ken was once approached by the son of one of the artists from the Ghost Army about his father's letters and photographs. The son wanted to give these items to the Museum of the Army and the World War II Museum, and Ken was to create the appraisal for these gifts for tax purposes.

Some famous names came out of the Ghost Army of WWII. Bill Blass, the fashion designer, is one, and Ellsworth Kelly (his painting is mentioned in Chapter 11) is another.

The Ghost Army is my final proof of art's power—even over the devastation of war.

THE GREAT IMPOSTER

But forgery can also morph into human pretense. One of my favorite examples is of General Tensor. Ken tells this story with a delicious German accent.

One day, Ken got a call from an insurance company about damaged items in a high-rise in New York City. A large painting with a heavy frame had fallen on a console table and smashed some expensive Meissen figures and other sculpture.

When Ken walked in, a man in his seventies (wearing a short-sleeved military shirt with two stars on the collar and a nametag that said TENSOR) greeted him impatiently. In the foyer behind him was a desk with a sign that said General Tensor.

In a heavy accent, he announced, "I don't need you here. Some others have been before to look at our broken pieces."

Ken responded, "But I am the art appraiser, the one who will determine the value of the items and what can be restored."

"I am very busy. I have a conference call soon with the Joint Chiefs of Staff, and I can't miss this call," General Tensor said with irritation.

"When is the conference?" asked Ken

"Three o'clock," snapped Tensor.

"I will be out of here way before then," Ken said, walking into the adjoining living room.

Ken began his work, taking pictures and notes about the damaged antiques. And Tensor followed him, intrigued.

Ken said, "I see how the picture fell and broke the vases, but where is the Meissen?"

"I sent it out to be repaired. But I have pictures." Tensor went back to his desk. He rummaged through it and then threw his pen down. He can't find the pictures. "I don't remember where we put them.

"I can't find them, but my wife knows where they are."

He picked up the phone, and said, "You must come home now. I need the pictures of the Meissen." Then he threw down the phone.

It was quite a collection of antiques. While Ken was working, Tensor brought in a framed invitation.

"Let me show you something," he said. "I fought in the Battle of Britain in 1941, and the Queen invited me to a reunion in 1960 to celebrate the pilots."

Ken looked at the elaborate script and nodded appreciatively.

This sharing broke the ice, and Ken felt free to ask how he collected so much fine art.

Tensor, loosened up now, said, "Most of these are from Wannsee, (the German town where much of the stolen Nazi art was stored). I mean my mother's house in Virggineeya."

Tensor then left and came back with the Meissen pictures, which he found in his desk.

"Have you ever been shot in the leg? It is very painful," said General Tensor.

Then he showed Ken a dagger with the inscription *Alles fier Deutschland* (All for Germany). Ken held the knife and nodded.

"Do you know why this is special? See the number one on the flange? It belonged to Ernst Rohm, the head of the brownshirts, the SA, which became the SS." (In the Night of the Long Knives, Rohm was strangled with a piano wire, for he was a threat to Hitler's supremacy.)

Ken finished his work, and as he was leaving, he asked, "Are you still on active duty?"

Tensor puffed out his chest, "Oh, yes. I have the Congressional Medal of Honor. *Und* all of us who hold this, must be on active duty."

Tensor rummaged in his desk again. The doorbell rang, and it was his wife. He opened the door about two inches, and Ken heard a heavily accented female voice say, "I come queek."

"I found them," Tensor shouted and slammed the door in his wife's face.

Then, he presented Ken with a document which said *Congressional Medal of Honor*. There was no medal, only a formal proclamation. It looks real, although Ken's suspicions were really simmering now.

Ken left the apartment. He had books at home which listed the recipients of the Congressional Medal of Honor from the Plains Wars in the 19th century to the Korean War.

Tensor's name was not in any of the listings. Then he called a friend in Washington and asked for his help.

After a day or two, his friend at the State Department gave him the lowdown. He said that Tensor was a Lieutenant in German intelligence, specializing in Russian matters. The US Army captured him after the war and made a deal.

"We will bring your belongings, including your art, to the US if you help us with intelligence." They made him a Sergeant in the Air Force.

Ken's friend said, "This guy has been known to masquerade as a general."

"Wow," Ken said. "What about his wife? She sounded Asian."

"She is—and a prostitute."

Later, Ken was assigned back to the Tensors by the insurance company. They wanted to verify the extensive repairs done on the paintings and the collection of small sculpture. Tensor had also made some claims on a coin collection which turned out to be fake.

This time, Ken was warmly ushered into a plain foyer, with the general in a simple tee shirt. No sign of any masquerade.

His wife came forward and said, "You famous man. I want to take with you peecture."

So, Ken posed with General Tensor's wife.

And Tensor asked one more German-centric question: "What kind of car do you drive?" asked Tensor.

"A 1975 Mercedes," Ken answered.

Tensor disappeared, then returned with his hand behind his back. Bringing his arm around, he handed Ken a round object, a little worn.

"Gas caps for Mercedes are hard to replace," Tensor said. "Take it as my gift."

The gas cap Tensor handed to Ken, the imposter's gift, was odd, but practical—even thoughtful. Someday, a careless gas station attendant will forget to put Ken's back on the tank, and Tensor's gift will be welcome.

Likewise, I hand this book to you as we part. Without knowing your very particular horrors, I feel like an imposter. Forgive that ignorance; only you know what you endure. But whatever part of your heart that is the glove compartment, I hope this souvenir will be tucked in there.

Eventually, may you find some bit of advice that will lift you out of grief, depression, self-pity, panic, loneliness, internet madness, doctor confusion, pain, thoughts of death, the hit-and-run tactics of guerilla reminders, and the traps of an illness identity that undermines your authentic self.

The stories of how appraisals are generated through the loss of art through death, debt, divorce, and disaster may remind you of your own legacy and how our attachment to things of beauty mirror our own culpability or grace: in the givers, the takers, the hoarders, the crooks—what Jimmy Baldwin called "the sons of bitches we are and the miracles we can be."

Above all, welcome the pleasures of acute simultaneity, the philosophical, psychological tonic of our recommended special blend: love enduring in the face of death. Pies, indeed, to die for. And don't forget, art is not a thing, but a way, a way of seeing and savoring. It can distract, delight, comfort, and fill in the blanks of our tattered lives.

Finally, pursue what thrills you, you the distinct spiritual and emotional self you have become, one enriched by this chapter of terror you are passing through, this valley before your second mountain. Celebrate that real you before it is too late.

We cannot make our lives longer, but we can make them wider, deeper, and higher.

APPENDIX 1
STRONG RECOMMENDATIONS

- Read Lissa Rankin, *Mind over Medicine.* Believe it!!!!
- Meditate and exercise the mind.
- Find the right doctors who appreciate your vitality, your fears, your passions.
- Develop compassion for others. Join a group that shares your interest in something apart from being cured of cancer: country music, antiques, books, travel, model trains. This will not only feed your mind but also provide you with the opportunity to know something of the lives of others, their challenges, and hopes. Find a project that helps others. Try hard to live an intention-driven life. Work with children, seniors, immigrants, the poor, recovering addicts, the chronically ill—all call to your abilities to lessen their burdens.
- Practice gentle but consistent exercise. The opposite of depression is motion. Acquire a healthy diet; stay abreast of medical breakthroughs from acclaimed cancer

treatment centers, especially advertising supplements; educate yourself on alternative treatments, such as on the website The Truth about Cancer. The list goes on and can make this period of your life a pretty full part-time job.

- Cultivate and pursue laughter, comedy. Build it into your day with programs, podcasts, films, certain friends.

- Surround yourself with beauty, wonder, awe—with art, music, travel, and magic. Start by deliberately bringing joy into your life with ordinary engines of happiness: color, shape, nature, movement, etc.

- Practice slowly facing death by first cultivating your beliefs in the supernatural. If you can, embrace the spirit plane through reincarnation, traditional concepts of the afterlife, quantum theory, or any other cultural bridge that encourages the notion that death is not necessarily an end. Who, after they passed, left you with a feeling that they're still around in some way? Do they help you in your daily life? Do they send you special dreams? Do you believe in angels? What is stopping you? What are your angels' names? If this approach seems ridiculous, study quantum theory and the notion that we are energy that cannot be destroyed and consider that we survive in some other plane.

- Plan your memorial service, so it's a celebration of your life. Think about cremation or burial, the location, the script, the music, the photographs. Will you have a video? Who will produce and direct the event? Write it all down.

- Develop an ability to tolerate and savor acute simultaneity, accepting the real possibility of death in the near future, as well as the wonder of life as you're living it now. It's a poignant and sharp taste in the brain, like the tang of a ripe, sour cherry. But it's also a wise lesson in reality. Most of life is a blend of the two ends of this spectrum: the thrill of your four-year-old grandson's voice on the phone, "Hi Glamma!" and the fact slapping against the joy: he is 3,000 miles away.

- Savor your husband's expression as he gazes at the sexy, young thirty-year-old walking by—and his half grin as he looks at you when he knows you have caught him at it. The applause you receive when you finish a talk on Art and Healing, and the enthusiastic compliment of the audience member when they congratulate you on "beating cancer," knowing you have not beaten it at all!

APPENDIX 2

WHAT I DO WHEN I AM FEELING LONELY, DEPRESSED, SCARED, OR PANICKED

*Everyone is after me
to stay positive, but
tonight I feel like
pissing on a rock.*

—Mark Nepo

- First, I meditate for five or ten minutes
- Call a girlfriend and tell her a story about angels, like this one: Yesterday, I left my purse in a shopping cart outside a store and drove away. When I stopped at the next errand, I realized it, and having my phone, I called the store and discovered the manager had found it and brought it into the cashier. It was waiting for me an hour later when I returned through heavy Christmas

traffic—everything exactly as I had left it—money, credit cards, glasses, calendar. A small miracle.

- Prepare to go out: write a note to my husband and put it on the kitchen cutting board next to the new mail, so he will see it when he comes in, something about liking a recipe in his favorite magazine, *Saveur*. I sign it with a big heart.

- Go to a scheduled physical therapy session—lots of stretching, some aerobics, and a fifteen-minute gentle massage. In the car, listen to a great book on Audible or a library CD. I plan a Christmas pizza gift for the staff when I'm not there the following week. In the car, I listen to a book on witchcraft that tells me that in the sixteenth century, witches were poor women living outside of town who were over forty. Remarkable: some of those women were not only scared of being burnt at the stake, but also had breast cancer! Take that for your "new normal."

I find a funny movie for watching later.

I remember that I am *not* the results of the blood tests, the PET scans, the MRIs. I widen my perspective. I am *not* merely a cancer patient. I am a dynamic grandma who has lots of friends, plans for the future, a great wardrobe, a writing and speaking career, and an intention to inspire, move, and entertain others. And I might be a faerie!

I watch a volunteer at the local church prepare for a holiday craft fair. I thank them for this colossal effort to help Saint Joan's.

I change my mindset by counting my blessings—the kids are well, my wonderful husband, the cruise we're taking in December to South America, the beautiful house we live in.

My friends. I call up one of them and organize a birthday lunch for another friend.

I plan my wardrobe for the next three holiday parties. *I have holiday parties in my life*, I tell myself. I remember that I have had a wonderful life. (Parties are out during COVID, but we can Zoom cocktails! And the top of you—up to your tits—can be glamorous!)

I watch the Truth About Cancer's new symposium and see the discoveries for cancer care and the way people with metastatic cancer are living longer. I start to read *The Cancer Revolution* or *Cancer: Step Outside of the Box.*

I project that my next visit to my oncologist will be uplifting and joyous . . . as it has been for the last four years.

Finally . . .

I call on my mom's spirit and Dad's to get me out of the funk. I have faith that I'll live as long as my mother did—91. She tells me this from the other side, in a dream, in a whisper. That means I have fifteen more years. I will see Mac Weaver drive a car. He will be turning eighteen. I will be with him in the front seat, my ninety-year-old hair just recently dyed blonde, a colorful scarf on my head as we head out in that red convertible. He grins into the wind on the Pacific Coast Highway. As we turn into the traffic, I look for somebody seeing us, someone who might say, "Look at that lucky old lady having fun!"

APPENDIX 3

THE QUICK RECIPE FOR TURNING AROUND A BAD DAY

- Yoga, physical exercise
- Meditation
- Connecting with others
- Planning for the future
- Gratitude
- Connecting with spirit
- Learning about healing in modern and holistic medicine
- Comedy; funny movies; a witty friend
- Note how you have survived thus far
- Compassion for others and an intention-driven life
- Loving gestures (random acts of kindness)
- Realize how mind is more powerful than any medicine
- Listening to your favorite musician playing his favorite music
- Finding your favorite painter, ceramicist, sculptor, collage expert, etc.

APPENDIX 4

READING LIST

Rick Beyer and Elizabeth Sayles, *The Ghost Army of World War II*

Ty Bollinger, *Cancer: Step Outside the Box, 6th Edition;* also, TheTruthAboutCancer.org

Alain de Botton and John Armstrong, *Art as Therapy*

Kate Bowler, *Everything Happens for a Reason and Other Lies I've Loved*; also podcast katecbowler.com

David Brooks, *The Second Mountain: The Quest for a Moral Life*

Bill Bryson, *The Body: A Guide for Occupants*

Laura Carfang, www.SurvivingBreastCancer.org

Leigh Erin Connealy, M.D., *The Cancer Revolution: A Groundbreaking Program to Reverse and Prevent Cancer*

Lynn Darling, "Is There a Cure for Loneliness," *AARP Magazine*, December 2019/January 2020, pp. 55-60

Colin Dickey, *Cranioklepty: Grave Robbing and the Search for Genius*

Robert D. Feder, Charles Rosoff, Aleza Tadri Friedman General
Editors, *Valuing Specific Assets in Divorce;* with a section
by Ken Linsner

Melinda Gates, *The Moment of Lift: How Empowering Women
Changes the World*

Gawande, Atul, *Being Mortal: Medicine and What Matters in
the End*

Adam Gopnik, *Winter: Five Windows on the Season*

Sari Harrar, "Happiness in Hard Times," *AARP: The Magazine,*
June/July 2020, p. 57

Leslie Jamieson: *NY Times Book Review,* "The Best Book She
Ever Got as a Present," September 19, 2019

Paul Joannides, *The Guide to Getting It On*

Paul Kalanithi, *When Breath Becomes Air*

Annie Lamott, *Almost Everything: Notes on Hope*

Ingrid Fetell Lee, *Joyful: The Surprising Power of Ordinary
Things to Create Extraordinary Happiness*

Anne Loeser, *The Insider's Guide to Metastatic Breast Cancer: A
Summary of the Disease and Its Treatment*

BJ Miller, *A Beginner's Guide to the End: Practical Advice for
Living Life and Facing Death*

Mukherjee, Siddhartha, *The Emperor of All Maladies: A
Biography of Cancer*

Mark Nepo, *The Book of Awakening: Having the Life You Want
by Being Present to the Life You Have*

Mark Nepo, *Inside the Miracle: Enduring Suffering, Approaching
Wholeness*

Mark Nepo and Richard Frankel, *Surviving Has Made Me
Crazy: Poems*

Lissa Rankin, *Mind over Medicine: Scientific Proof that You Can
Heal Yourself*

Keith Richards with James Fox, *LIFE*

Phakyab Rinpoche and Sofia Stril-Rever, *Meditation Saved My Life: A Tibetan Lama and the Healing Power of the Mind*

Bob Roth, *Strength in Stillness: The Power of Transcendental Meditation*

Andrew Schulman, *Waking the Spirit: A Musician's Journey Healing Body, Mind and Soul*

Dr. Kenneth Silvestri, *A Wider Lens: How to See Your Life Differently*

Nate Staniforth, *Here Is Real Magic: A Magician's Search for Wonder in the Modern World*

Melanie Thernstrom, *The Pain Chronicles: Cures, Myths, Mysteries, Prayers, Diaries, Brain Scans, Healing, and the Science of Suffering*

Kelly A. Turner, Remission: *Surviving Cancer Against All Odds*

Patricia Vigderman, *Possibility: Essays against Despair*

Chris Wark, *Chris Survived Cancer: A Comprehensive Plan for Healing Naturally*

Gary Zukav, *The Seat of the Soul, 25th edition*

APPENDIX 5
QUESTIONS FOR GROUP DISCUSSION

CHAPTER 1: GRIEF

- What do you know about the mother's (who lost her son through suicide) grief, based on her posture of being in the walker and her incessant talking?
- My cousin lost her fifty-two-year-old daughter to a heart condition. She's become obsessed with Facebook posts since then. What other ways do we cope with losing a loved one; the diagnosis of a terminal disease; the loss of a job?
- What do you say to a friend who is clearly in grief? (See Kate Bowler's, *Everything Happens for a Reason,* pp. 173-175)
- Share how you managed to overcome a period of grief. How long did it take you to return to some kind of normalcy? What activities helped get you there?

- What book would you recommend to anyone enduring grief?
- Do you agree that hoarding is a kind of hyper-response to grief for the material? What other motives may be behind hoarding?
- Write an ending to the banker's story? What *is* behind the door of his "mother's room?" Who discovers this?

CHAPTER 2: SELF-PITY

- Choose an artist you love and discover his life story. What does it tell you?
- When have you felt most compassionate in the last week or so? What situation made you feel this emotion? Did some action follow from this emotion?
- What's the difference between empathy and compassion?
- Have you experienced what Mark Nepo calls a "lift?" This emotion, this change in perspective, takes us out of our self-pity and reminds us that we are *not* simply a wound, an illness, a loss.

CHAPTER 3: DEPRESSION

- Which of the "solutions" have worked for you in the past? What are you exploring now if you sometimes experience depression?
- What has been your experience with depression during the Coronavirus period?
- How has travel impacted your frame of mind?
- What role does physical action play in banishing depression?

CHAPTER 4: PANIC ATTACKS

- Panic can last a few moments, an hour or longer. Can you remember when you last had a panic attack and what triggered it?
- Which of the solutions do you think is most helpful?
- Discuss Dr. Turner's list of remission factors. Which of these needs more explanation? Which was most surprising?
- Will you share a favorite daydream? (please refrain from X-rated choices), one that always brings a smile to your heart.

Discuss the difference between a panic attack and heart attack

More likely a panic attack	More likely a heart attack
Sudden onset with extreme stress	Sudden onset, onset during physical exertion, or sharp stabbing pain in the chest on awakening
Pain in the middle of the chest	Squeezing pain and pressure in the chest
Pain that improves over time	Pain radiating to arm, jaw, shoulder, neck
Racing heart, shakiness, tingling hands	Pain that worsens over time
Symptoms that resolve within thirty minutes	Nausea and vomiting
A history of anxiety and worry	Longer lasting symptoms
	Personal or family history of heart related factors

CHAPTER 5: BATTLING LONELINESS

- What other support groups have you found online, in person, and in your region? What have been the advantages of participating?
- Kate Bowler talks about the loneliness she felt as a new parent. Comment on that experience.
- What is meant by the statement: We need not only to be in the company of people, but also to be *known*.
- And what of Jane's choices for beneficiaries? What do you think of these? Have you thought of your legacy? What, apart from money and property, would you leave to your family, friends, and chosen philanthropies?

CHAPTER 6: INTIMACY PROBLEMS

- What's your reaction to the discussion of sexuality in the context of such serious health concerns? Does it really matter?
- How much does age play a part?
- How do friendships, like yours, change when a friend has a frightening diagnosis?
- Do you think Subash "inherited" his father's criminality?

CHAPTER 7: INFORMATION OVERLOAD

- Take a look at TheTruthAboutCancer.org and offer your impression of the site.
- Offer an example of a "fake news" cancer cure you discovered on the internet.

- Have you thought about selling a work of art you own? How would you go about it?
- Do you consider art an investment?

CHAPTER 8: DOCTORS

- Our culture has traditionally held doctors in high esteem. Do you feel that way? Can you describe a "good" doctor you've known—and his or her opposite? What are the salient differences?
- Explore Ancestry.com or focus on one relative who intrigues you. Find out as much as you can about him or her.
- What or who fascinates you and why?
- Do your discovered ancestors tell you anything about yourself you didn't know?

CHAPTER 9: PAIN

- What pain remedies have you experienced yourself?
- How have you helped someone else in pain?
- Do you know anyone who became addicted to pain medication?
- What's your reaction to Imelda Marcos' solutions to insomnia?

CHAPTER 10: THOUGHTS OF DEATH

- What steps have you taken to provide for your own transition: Long term care insurance, an estate plan,

Power of Attorney, instructions on treatment, Living Will, funeral arrangements?

- What are your beliefs in the afterlife? The power of prayer?
- Do you believe our deceased loved ones are somehow still with us?
- What about magic?
- Has an experience of wonder ever felt as if it had a physical effect on you? Can you describe it?

CHAPTER 11: GUERILLA ATTACKS

- Give an example of a guerilla attack that recently stunned you.
- What did you do about it?
- When was the last time you looked at old photographs? Which ones made you feel good about your history?

CHAPTER 12: GETTING STUCK IN A CANCER IDENTITY

- Who do you know who exudes confidence?
- Which of the book collectors do you identify with?
- Tell us about an experience of the sublime.
- When have you felt caught in the trap of "a cancer patient?"
- Authenticity: Why is it important? How do you achieve it?

ACKNOWLEDGMENTS

Ken is not only a major character in the book; he is the living, breathing reason I could write it. The setting, the resources, the time were his gifts to me. Also, I have gratefully garnered the stories about his clients and art losses, and *Pies to Die For* would not exist without Ken's expertise and remarkable memory.

As a sixties rock-and-roller, I recall Keith Richards, guitar player and composer of the Rolling Stones, and his salute to the brilliant drum beat of Charlie Watts: "Its rhythm," said Keith, is "the bed I lie on, musically me and Charlie." This book, our marriage, is the "bed I lie on, musically me and Ken." Thank you, my darling

I salute my doctors for keeping me alive through faith, skill, expertise, patience, and creativity. Most of all, I thank them for believing in me and my inner pilot.

Thanks to the authors I have read. Truly, the books cited in the Reading List have been my guides and inspiration in greater understanding of health, philosophy, psychology, mental acumen, history, humanity, and transformation. Especially authors Lissa Rankin, Leslie Jamieson, David Brooks, Joy Ingrid Fetell, Anne Lamott, Ty Bolinger, Kelly Turner, Ken Silvestri and others—all have been in the room where it happened. I'm so grateful for their work.

Thank you to Nancy Erickson and my book-writing mastermind group. This work would not exist without the steady guidance and encouragement of my teacher, editor, and publisher, Nancy. She is so clearly an example of an authentic power because her personality expresses her soul's desire—to improve the world through the message of those who would help others. And I was lifted up and kept on track with the work of Linda, Heather, and Teresa. Their struggles mirrored my own, and so I was ravenous for their responses to my words. A feast after a tough week! Thank you for creating parallel universes. I could look at your faces to see my own. And, therefore, kept going.

Friends, beta readers, believers in me: Thank you for work on the cover design: Don Blauweiss, Maureen Bryant, and Laura Carfang. And to Lynn Maier and Sheila Pearl for early readings of the manuscript. Also for heart and soul support: Marianne Carroll, Monique Caubere, Diane Dudzinski, Violette Essman, Allen Goldberg, Tracey Lawrence, Vince McKewin, Mary Sturm, Natasha Rabin, Doreen Rhodes, Holly Whitstock Seeger, Ken Silvestri.

ABOUT THE AUTHOR

Carole Weaver, PhD, is a writer, professional speaker, and fund-raising consultant who lives in Rockland County, New York, with her husband, Ken, an international art appraiser and conservator. She has written *Side Effects: The Art of Surviving Cancer* (2016) and, as Cat Weaver, she is a co-writer with Ken Silvestri and Natasha Rabin, in *Train Romance*, a collection of poetry and photographs. *Pies to Die For* traces her diagnosis of metastatic cancer and remarkable continuing journey since 2016. Her two sons, James and David, live in California, and so does her grandson, Mac Weaver, now five years old.

Made in the USA
Columbia, SC
25 May 2021